Chart of Accounts for HOSPITALS

L. VANN SEAWELL

An Accounting & Reporting Reference Guide

HFMA® HEALTHCARE FINANCIAL MANAGEMENT ASSOCIATION

A HEALTHCARE 2000 PUBLICATION

PROBUS PUBLISHING
Chicago, Illinois
Cambridge, England

A HEALTHCARE 2000 PUBLICATION

ISBN 1-55738-619-6

Printed in the United States of America

BB

1 2 3 4 5 6 7 8 9 0

RR/BJS

Table of Contents

Foreword

It is widely recognized that information is the key to power. However, sometimes overlooked is the necessity that information be properly organized in order to fulfill this potential. A chart of accounts is the framework for organizing financial information. Thus, this chart of accounts provides a framework for making financial information about hospitals useful.

Dr. Vann Seawell has been the pioneer and guiding force in preparation of charts of accounts for hospitals, developing the groundbreaking American Hospital Association (AHA) chart in 1966. The chart of accounts has been periodically updated, but a great deal has happened in hospital operations and in financial information since this chart was last updated. Therefore, this chart moves the framework for organizing financial information by hospitals into the present with a structure for the future.

As the Healthcare Financial Management Association undertook a project to update and reissue this fundamental tool for hospital financial management, it made two essential decisions that have far-reaching impact. One, they persuaded Dr. Seawell to accept the challenge of designing a chart of accounts that recognizes current and future needs. And, the HFMA committed to a series of charts of accounts, with the chart for hospitals setting the standard. While there have been charts of accounts for hospitals in the past, other sectors of the healthcare industry have had less well-developed guidelines or no guidelines at all. As the range of institutions involved with healthcare have grown, the need to provide specific assistance has become more apparent, and this chart of accounts launches the project to meet more fully the needs of the industry.

It has been a pleasure to work with Dr. Seawell on this exciting endeavor. Rich Telkamp and Bill Titera have provided invaluable assistance along with many others who provided essential information and reviewed material at critical times.

Hospital financial mangers will find this chart provides the framework for organizing financial information to meet current needs. Financial managers in other sectors of the healthcare industry can look forward to similar assistance in the near future.

Ronald R. Kovener, CAE
President, Association Information Management Service, Inc.
Former President, HFMA

1

Introduction

1.1 The contemporary hospital is a remarkably complex organization of specialized resources whose administration is one of the most difficult applications of the management art. Hospitals must make available on a virtually continuous basis an ever-expanding range of services. Most of these healthcare services are provided by highly skilled personnel in a diversity of professions and require substantial investments in plant and equipment.

1.2 The social, economic, scientific, and technological changes of the last several decades have greatly complicated hospital management. They also have made accounting, as an information system, an even more vital and integral part of the management process. The development of new and better methods of accumulating and communicating quantitative data relating to the operating results and financial position of hospitals has become an imperative in the healthcare industry. Even greater emphasis also must be given to an intelligent interpretation and utilization of the information generated by the accounting process.

1.3 Accounting is an essential management activity in all economic entities, regardless of type or size. A principal purpose of accounting is to provide useful financial information about an entity's activities and affairs. This information is intended primarily for use in decision making by the management of the entity. In addition, the information is important to the needs of various external users such as investors, creditors, other resource providers, governmental agencies, and the general public.

1.4 These decisions directly affect the manner in which limited resources are allocated to, and employed in, individual entities. As a result, the information generated by the accounting process plays a significant role in determining the types and quantities of products and services that are produced and consumed. The recording and reporting of reliable financial information relevant to users' needs clearly must be viewed as a function of extreme importance in the economy.

1.5 This book is the first of a planned series of publications concerned with charts of accounts (and related accounting issues) for various types of healthcare provider organizations. The healthcare entity to which this book is directed is the hospital enterprise organized and operated either on a not-for-profit or investor-owned basis.

Hospital managers and interested external parties are more heavily dependent than ever before upon the information provided by the accounting process. It is clear that the effectiveness of decision making by internal and external users is directly related to the quality of the information made available to them. The major objective of this book is to provide guidance that will assist hospitals in their continuing efforts to develop financial information of the highest possible quality. The required qualitative characteristics of this information are described in Chapter 2, starting at paragraph 6.

HOSPITAL ORGANIZATION

1.6 Regardless of the type of ownership, the essential function and primary objective of the hospital is the provision of quality healthcare services at reasonable costs. A hospital also may be involved in medical research and educational programs. In carrying out its mission, the hospital employs many different types of human, physical, and financial resources. A well-conceived plan of organization must be established and maintained if these resources are to be utilized effectively.

1.7 The activities of any enterprise must be divided into manageable units, and organized into a coordinated and cooperative effort, to achieve its objectives. For management and accounting purposes, it is essential that clear lines of authority and clear definitions of responsibilities be established. Principles of organization such as "unity of command"—an individual should be responsible to only one person —and "span of control"—no manager should be responsible for the direct supervision of the work of an excessive number of subordinates—should be observed in devising the organization plan.

1.8 A hospital's organizational structure generally is depicted in a formal organization chart such as the one presented in Figure 1-1. (The important relationship between the organization structure and the chart of accounts is described in Chapter 4, starting at paragraph 4.18.)[1] This chart is illustrative only; it should not be regarded as a recommended pattern of organization. No two hospitals are, or should be, organized in exactly the same way. Differing organizational structures exist because of differences in hospital size, range of services, management style, personnel capabilities, and other factors. As a result, there is no single plan of organization that is applicable to all hospitals.

1.9 At the top of the organization chart is the hospital's governing board (usually called the "board of directors" or "board of trustees"). Ultimate authority and responsibility for the prudent management of the hospital's resources and operations rests with the board. Its members formulate general objectives and broad policies, approve budgets, and monitor the hospital's activities. The board, how-

1 Paragraphs 4.18 through 4.22 discuss the relationship between the hospital organization chart and the chart of accounts. Figure 4-4 indicates specific account numbers for the pharmacy and housekeeping departments as illustrations of this relationship.

ever, does not directly manage the day-to-day business of the hospital; this authority is delegated to the chief executive officer ("president" or "administrator"). Authority for medical and surgical services is delegated to a physician (often called the "medical director" or "chief of medical staff"). The president and the medical director, because their responsibilities are interrelated, must work always in close cooperation.

1.10 It is impossible, even in small hospitals, for the chief executive officer to exercise continuous and direct personal supervision over all hospital activities. As shown in Figure 1-1, hospital activities usually are organized into major divisional units such as nursing services, other professional services, general services, and fiscal and administrative services. Each divisional unit is headed by an individual (director or vice president) to whom the chief executive officer delegates authority for managing its operations. Divisional directors are responsible to the chief executive officer who, in turn, is responsible to the board of directors.

1.11 Each division is divided into subordinate organizational units (nursing units, departments) having a designated manager whose authority comes from the divisional director to whom he or she is responsible. In some cases, departments are organized into two or more sections, each of which is managed by a person responsible to the departmental manager.

1.12 Thus, the hospital entity is composed of organizational units. Each unit is a *responsibility center*. The individual in charge of each responsibility center is given the authority, within prescribed policies and practices, to take actions and make decisions necessary to effective management of the activities of the center. With such authority, that individual accepts responsibility for the achievement of the center's established objectives.

1.13 All responsibility centers incur expenses; some responsibility centers also generate revenues. Centers that do not generate revenues are referred to as *expense centers* or *cost centers*. (They also may be called *overhead*, or *support, centers*.) Those centers that generate revenues are called *revenue centers* or *profit centers*. In a *responsibility accounting system*, expenses are recorded and reported according to the centers responsible for the incurrence of the expenses; revenues are recorded and reported according to the centers whose activities produced the revenues. The classification of revenues and expenses by responsibility center facilitates the process of managerial planning and control.

1.14 The manner in which the chart (classification) of accounts is directly linked to the organization structure is described in Chapter 4 (starting at paragraph 4.18). In a few states (as in California), a uniform chart of accounts is mandated by law. Internal managerial needs, however, may not be appropriately met by a chart of accounts mandated by an external authority. The position taken in this book is that each hospital should construct its chart of accounts to conform to its own particular organizational pattern, thereby ensuring that informational requirements of its management are given priority. In designing the chart of accounts, however, the needs of external information users certainly must be considered, but they are secondary considerations.

Figure 1–1
Hospital Organization Chart

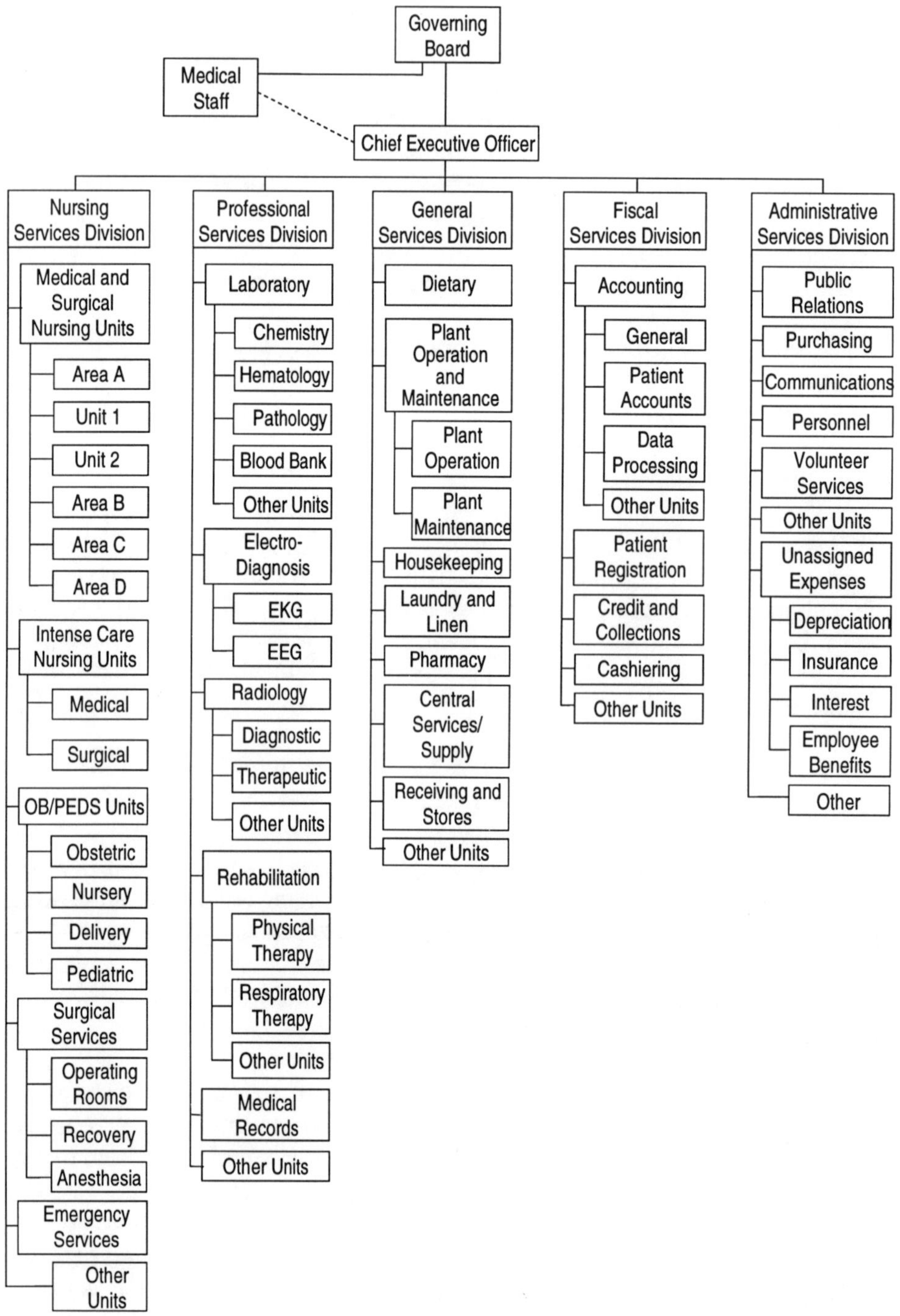

MANAGERIAL NEED FOR INFORMATION

1.15 Within any enterprise, there is an imperative need for statistical and financial information. This is particularly true of hospitals due to the large number of individual, yet interdependent, responsibility centers whose activities must be planned and controlled.

1.16 Effective management of the hospital requires that the objectives of each responsibility center be clearly established. These objectives initially may be expressed in statistical terms such as hours of nursing care, number of laboratory examinations, and pounds of laundry. Measurements of expected service volume then can be translated into monetary terms such as anticipated dollars of expenditures and revenues. These level-of-activity and financial objectives are coordinated into an overall operating plan (budget) for the hospital as a whole. Budgets usually are developed for a one-year period, and broken down into monthly segments. (In some hospitals, the calendar year is broken down into 13 budgetary and reporting periods of four weeks each.) The monthly budgeted amounts, however, are not simply one-twelfth of the annual budgeted amounts; the monthly budgets of revenues and expenses should reflect the amounts that management expects to be earned or incurred in each month.

1.17 As the year progresses, each month's actual results (revenues and expenses) are compared with budgeted objectives so that the performance of each responsibility center can be evaluated by department managers, by divisional directors, by the chief executive officer, and by the board of directors. Variances from budgeted objectives should be closely monitored. Where, within the hospital, do significant variances appear? Why have the variances occurred? Who is responsible? What corrective actions should be taken? Answers to these questions permit intelligent decisions to be made to ensure that the variances do not recur in the future.

1.18 It is in this way that hospital management utilizes statistical and financial information, both historical and projected. Such information is essential to managerial planning and control. To be useful, however, the information must be relevant to the needs of hospital managers. This is why the classifications used in recording and reporting revenues and expenses should conform to the organizational structure of the hospital.

1.19 The effectiveness of the management functions of establishing objectives, planning, and controlling therefore depends largely upon:

1. The existence of a sound organizational structure, and

2. The accumulation and communication of relevant and reliable financial and statistical information relating to each area responsibility within the hospital.

The effort expended in the production of reliable and relevant information, however, is largely wasted unless governing boards and hospital managers at all levels are willing and able to use that information. They must have both an understanding of the information and an appreciation of its value to the management process.

THE ACCOUNTING FUNCTION

1.20 The hospital accounting function, simply stated, is to provide useful information about the hospital's activities and affairs. This information is of a statistical and financial character; it is both historical and projected in nature. As noted earlier, the information is essential to effective management of the hospital; it also is useful in decision making by parties external to the hospital. The most important use of financial and related statistical information, however, is in managerial planning and control.

1.21 Hospital accounting is defined as the accumulation, communication, and interpretation of historical and projected economic data relating to the financial position and operating results of a hospital enterprise, for purposes of decision making by its management and by various external parties.

1.22 The term *accumulation* refers to the process of recording the business transactions and financial events that occur in the economic life of the hospital. Central to the recording process is the use of a data classification system (a "chart of accounts") that is designed to produce useful information about the hospital's resources, obligations, revenues, and expenses. (An illustrative chart of accounts is described in Chapters 4, 5, and 6 of this book.) It should be emphasized, however, that both monetary and statistical data must be considered concurrently in any analysis, evaluation, or interpretation.

1.23 *Communication* is the reporting of recorded information to users of that information. This is accomplished by the issuance of accounting reports and financial statements such as income statements and balance sheets. For internal management purposes, revenues and expenses should be reported in the same responsibility center classifications employed in the recording process. This classification system, however, may not be appropriate for external reporting purposes. The informational needs of management are paramount, but the requirements of external users also must be considered in the design of the chart of accounts. Illustrative financial statements, based upon the chart of accounts outlined in Chapter 4, are provided in Chapter 7 of this book.

1.24 The word *interpretation* refers to the analysis and evaluation of reported information for decision-making purposes. It is not enough merely to record and to report; the accounting responsibility extends to the function of assisting users in the interpretation of reported data. This is necessary if users are to comprehend fully the significance of the information and to utilize it in an intelligent manner.

INTERNAL CONTROL

1.25 The reliability of information generated by the accounting process depends largely upon an effective system of internal control. Internal control has been defined as follows:

> A process, effected by an entity's board of directors, management, or other personnel, designed to provide reasonable assurance regarding the achievement of objectives in the following categories: (1) effectiveness and efficiency of operations, (2) reliability of financial reporting, and (3) compliance with applicable laws and regulations.[2]

The Auditing Standards Board has indicated that the broad objective of internal accounting control is to provide management with reasonable, but not absolute, assurance that assets are safeguarded from unauthorized use or disposition and that financial records are maintained in a manner to permit the preparation of reliable financial statements.[3] This objective can be realized if:

- Transactions are executed in accordance with management's general or specific authorization,
- Transactions are recorded in conformity with generally accepted accounting principles,
- Accountability for assets is maintained,
- Access to assets is permitted only in accordance with management authorization, and
- Asset records are compared with existing assets at reasonable intervals, with appropriate action being taken with respect to any differences.

In Statement of Auditing Standards (SAS) No. 55, an entity's internal control structure is defined to consist of the policies and procedures needed to provide reasonable assurance that the entity's objectives are achieved.[4] The elements of the structure include the accounting system, the control environment, control procedures, and management's decision-making process.

1.26 The components of internal control are set forth in a report issued by the Committee of Sponsoring Organizations of the Treadway Commission as follows:[5]

2 *Internal Control - Integrated Framework* (New York: Committee of Sponsoring Organizations of the Treadway Commission, 1992), p. 2.

3 Statement on Auditing Standards No. 30, *Reporting on Internal Accounting Control* (New York: AICPA, 1980).

4 Statement on Auditing Standards No. 55, *Consideration of the Internal Control Structure in a Financial Statement Audit* (New York: AICPA, 1988).

- *Control Environment.* The control environment sets the tone of an organization, influencing the control consciousness of its people. It provides a foundation for the other components of internal control, providing discipline and structure. Control-environment factors include the integrity, ethical values and competence of the entity's people; management's philosophy and operating style; the way management assigns authority and responsibility and organizes and develops its people; and the attention and direction provided by the board of directors.

- *Risk Assessment.* Every entity faces a variety of risks from external and internal sources that must be assessed. A precondition to risk assessment is establishment of objectives, linked at different levels and internally consistent. Risk assessment involves identification and analysis of relevant risks to achievement of the objectives, as a basis for determining how the risks should be managed. Because economic, industry, regulatory, and operating conditions will continue to change, mechanisms are needed to identify and deal with the special risks associated with change.

- *Control Activities.* Control activities encompass the policies and implementation procedures that help ensure management directives are effected. They help assure that necessary actions are taken to address risks to achievement of the entity's objectives. Control activities occur throughout the organization, at all levels and in all functions. They include a range of activities as diverse as approvals, authorizations, verifications, reconciliations, reviews of operating performance, security of assets, and segregation of duties.

- *Information and Communication.* Pertinent information must be identified and communicated to people in a form and time frame that enable them to carry out their responsibilities. Information systems produce the reports, containing operational, financial, and compliance-related information, that make it possible to run and control the business. They deal not only with internally generated data, but also information about external events, activities, and conditions necessary to informed business decision making and external reporting. Effective communication also must occur in a broader sense down, across, and up the organization. All personnel must receive a clear message from top management that control responsibilities must be taken seriously. They must understand their own role in the internal control system, as well as how individual activities relate to the work of others. And, they must have a means of communicating significant information upstream. There also needs to be effective communication with external parties: customers, suppliers, regulators, shareholders, and others.

5 *Internal Control - Integrated Framework* (New York: Committee of Sponsoring Organizations of the Treadway Commission, 1992), pp. 2-3.

- *Monitoring*. Internal control systems need to be monitored, a process that assesses the quality of the system's performance over time. This is accomplished through ongoing monitoring activities, separate evaluations, or a combination of the two. Ongoing monitoring occurs in the course of operations. It includes regular management and supervisory activities, and other actions personnel take in performing their duties. The scope and frequency of separate evaluations will depend primarily on an assessment of risks and the effectiveness of ongoing monitoring procedures. Internal control deficiencies should be reported upstream, with serious matters reported to top management and the board.

This view of internal control is a broad one, focusing on the fact that internal control is a process used to achieve all of the objectives of an enterprise: operations, financial reporting, and compliance.

2

Financial Accounting and Reporting Concepts

2.1 The Financial Accounting Standards Board (FASB) has issued a series of Statements of Financial Accounting Concepts (SFACs) whose major purpose is to provide the conceptual framework or theoretical foundation upon which financial accounting and reporting standards are to be based. Unlike the FASB Statements of Financial Accounting Standards (SFASs), SFACs do not establish generally accepted accounting principles (GAAP). They are intended, instead, to set forth a logical, consistent, and cohesive body of interrelated fundamental concepts to be used by the FASB in evaluating existing standards and developing new standards.

2.2 This chapter consists mainly of a brief summary of the financial accounting and reporting concepts that have been identified in SFACs issued by the FASB. The reader is urged to refer to the SFACs in their complete published form to secure a more complete understanding of the concepts. Materials that specifically relate to governmental hospitals are drawn from publications of the Governmental Accounting Standards Board (GASB).

OBJECTIVES OF FINANCIAL REPORTING

2.3 SFAC No. 1 establishes the objectives of general-purpose, external financial reporting by business enterprises. It is not applicable to internal reporting, but recognition is given to the fact that management is as interested in financial information as are external users. The stated objectives are that financial reporting should:[1]

1. Provide information that is useful to present and potential investors, creditors, and other users in making rational investment, credit, and similar decisions, assuming that users have a reasonable understanding of business activities and that users are willing to study the information with reasonable diligence,

2. Provide information to help present and potential investors, creditors, and other users in assessing the amounts, timing, and uncertainty of prospective net cash inflows to the enterprise, and

3. Provide information about the economic resources of the enterprise, the claims to those resources, and the effects of transactions or events that change its resources and claims against them.

The reported information should enable users to assess the performance of an enterprise in terms of earnings, cash flows, economic resources and obligations, and other factors that may affect its liquidity and solvency. Financial reporting should include explanations and interpretations by management to enhance the understandability and usefulness of the financial information provided.

2.4 SFAC No. 4 establishes the objectives of general purpose external financial reporting by not-for-profit organizations. The stated objectives are that financial reporting by such organizations should:[2]

1. Provide information that is useful to present and potential resource providers and other users in making rational decisions about the allocation of resources to those organizations;

2. Provide information to help present and potential resource providers and other users in assessing the services that the organization provides and its ability to continue to provide those services;

3. Provide information that is useful to present and potential resource providers and other users in assessing how managers of the organization have discharged their stewardship responsibilities, and about other aspects of their performance;

1 Statement of Financial Accounting Concepts No. 1, *Objectives of Financial Reporting by Business Enterprises* (Norwalk, Connecticut: FASB, 1978).

2 Statement of Financial Accounting Concepts No. 4, *Objectives of Financial Reporting by Nonbusiness Organizations* (Norwalk, Connecticut: FASB, 1980). The term "nonbusiness" has since been abandoned by the FASB in favor or "not-for-profit.

4. Provide information about the economic resources, obligations, and net resources of the organization, and the effects of transactions and events that change resources and interests in those resources;

5. Provide information about the performance of the organization during the reporting period;

6. Provide information about how the organization obtains and spends cash or other liquid resources, about its borrowings and repayment of borrowings, and about other factors that may affect the organization's liquidity; and

7. Include explanations and interpretations to help users understand the financial information provided.

Although not-for-profit hospitals generally have taken the position that they are *not* the type of organizations referred to by SFAC No. 4, these seven objectives would seem to be generally applicable to hospitals of all types.

2.5 The objectives of governmental financial reporting (including financial reporting by governmental hospitals) have been enumerated by the GASB as follows:[3]

1. Financial reporting should assist in fulfilling government's duty to be publicly accountable and should enable users to assess that accountability.

    a. Financial reporting should provide information to determine whether current-year revenues were sufficient to pay for current-year services.

    b. Financial reporting should demonstrate whether resources were obtained and used in accordance with the entity's legally adopted budget; it should also demonstrate compliance with other finance-related legal or contractual requirements.

    c. Financial reporting should provide information to assist users in assessing the service efforts, costs, and accomplishments of the governmental entity.

2. Financial reporting should assist users in evaluating the operating results of the governmental entity for the year.

    a. Financial reporting should provide information about sources and uses of financial resources.

3 *Codification of Governmental Accounting and Financial Reporting Standards* (Norwalk, Connecticut: GASB, 1990), Section 100, par. 177-179.

   b. Financial reporting should provide information about how the governmental entity financed its activities and met its cash requirements.

   c. Financial reporting should provide information necessary to determine whether the entity's financial position improved or deteriorated as a result of the year's operations.

3. Financial reporting should assist users in assessing the level of services that can be provided by the governmental entity and its ability to meet its obligations as they come due.

   a. Financial reporting should provide information about the financial position and condition of a governmental entity.

   b. Financial reporting should provide information about a governmental entity's physical and other nonfinancial resources having useful lives that extend beyond the current year, including information that can be used to assess the service potential of those resources.

   c. Financial reporting should disclose legal or contractual restrictions on resources and risks of potential loss of resources.

The similarities between these GASB financial reporting objectives and the FASB financial reporting objectives (investor-owned and not-for profit) are evident; users of general-purpose, external financial reports, whatever the nature of the reporting entity, need essentially the same information.

QUALITATIVE CHARACTERISTICS OF ACCOUNTING INFORMATION

2.6 SFAC No. 2 identifies the qualitative characteristics of accounting (financial) information that makes that information most meaningful and useful to users.[4] The two most important qualities of the information provided by financial reporting are *relevance* and *reliability*. Each of these qualities has three basic components.

Relevance

2.7 To be relevant to users, accounting information must be capable of making a difference in decision making by assisting users in predicting the outcomes of past, present, and future events, or in confirming or changing earlier expectations. The principal components of relevance are:

4 Statement of Financial Accounting Concepts No. 2, *Qualitative Characteristics of Accounting Information* (Norwalk, Connecticut: FASB, 1980).

1. *Predictive Value.* The quality of information that helps users to increase the likelihood of correctly forecasting the outcome of past or present events.

2. *Feedback Value.* The quality of information that enables users to confirm or correct prior expectations.

3. *Timeliness.* Having information available to a decision-maker before it loses its capacity to influence decisions.

Reliability

2.8 Reliability is the quality of information that assures the user that the information is reasonably free from error and bias, and faithfully represents what it purports to represent. The three principal components of reliability are:

1. *Verifiability.* The ability through consensus among measurers to ensure that information represents what it purports to represent, or that the chosen measurement method has been used without error or bias. (Bias in accounting measures means a tendency to be consistently too high or too low.)

2. *Representational Faithfulness.* Correspondence or agreement between a measure or description and the phenomenon that it purports to represent.

3. *Neutrality.* Absence in reported information of bias intended to attain a predetermined result or to induce a particular mode of behavior.

Other Qualities and Constraints

2.9 Closely related to relevance and reliability are certain other necessary qualitative characteristics of accounting information:

1. *Understandability.* The quality of information that enables users to perceive its significance. (It is assumed that users have a reasonable understanding of business activities, and are willing to study the information with reasonable diligence.)

2. *Comparability.* The quality of information that enables users to identify similarities in and differences between two sets of economic phenomena. (Comparability is enhanced by consistency: conformity from period to period with unchanged policies and practices.)

3. *Completeness.* The inclusion in reported information of everything material that is necessary for faithful representation of the relevant phenomena.

2.10 While it is desirable for accounting information to possess all qualitative characteristics described above, certain of the characteristics may not always be compatible. There may be times when one characteristic can be secured only by sacrificing another. As a result, trade-offs must be made on the basis of the relative importance of the characteristics that are involved.

2.11 Attainment of the desired qualitative characteristics of accounting information also is subject to other constraints:

1. *Materiality*. SFAC 2 defines materiality as "the magnitude of an omission or misstatement of accounting information that in the light of surrounding circumstances, makes it probable that the judgment of a reasonable person relying on the information would have been changed or influenced by the omission or misstatement." Materiality is an elusive concept whose appropriate application to a particular item of accounting information requires a judgment based upon the relative size of the item, the nature of the item, and other considerations. SFAC 2 provides no general standards for determining materiality.

2. *Costs and Benefits*. Accounting information provides certain benefits to users. The value of these benefits should be weighed against the costs of providing and using the information. If the costs exceed the benefits, the information has no net value and generally should not be provided. It is extremely difficult (if not impossible), however, to quantify the value of the benefits to users of accounting information. As a result, application of the pervasive cost/benefits restraint requires judgment.

2.12 The convention of *conservatism* is defined in SFAC 2 as "a prudent reaction to uncertainty to try to ensure that uncertainty and risks inherent in business situations are adequately considered." Historically, the providers and users of accounting information have generally preferred that possible errors in measurement be in the direction of understatement rather than overstatement of net income and net assets. This led to the notion that deliberate understatement is a virtue. It is not. There is a place for conservatism (meaning "prudence") in financial reporting, but the aim should be that of putting users in the best possible position to form their own opinions of the probable outcome of the events reported.

RECOGNITION AND MEASUREMENT IN FINANCIAL STATEMENTS

2.13 SFAC 5 provides recognition criteria and guidance as to what information should be included in financial statements and when. It also addresses certain measurement issues that are related to recognition.[5]

5 Statement of Financial Accounting Concepts No. 5, *Recognition and Measurement in Financial Statements of Business Enterprises* (Norwalk, Connecticut: FASB, 1984).

Financial Statements

2.14 Financial statements are the principal means of communicating useful financial information to external users. Certain information, however, is better provided (or can only be provided) by notes to the financial statements, by supplementary information, or by other means. These disclosures, amplifications, and explanations are essential to an understanding of the information recognized in financial statements, and are viewed as an integral part of them.

2.15 As discussed earlier in this chapter, SFAC 1 sets forth the objectives of financial reporting, and also indicates the kinds of information that financial reporting (including financial statements) should provide. Because of the large amount and wide variety of the information to be provided, several financial statements are required. A full set of financial statements for a period should include the following:

- Financial position at the end of the period (balance sheet).
- Earnings for the period (income statement).
- Comprehensive income (total nonowner changes in equity) for the period.
- Cash flows during the period (statement of cash flows).
- Investments by and distributions to owners during the period. (Not applicable to not-for-profit organizations.)

SFAC 5 did not provide guidelines as to the manner in which the above information should be displayed, but the FASB subsequently issued its Statement of Financial Accounting Standards No. 117 which provides the necessary guidelines for the financial statements of not-for-profit organizations.[6] The requirements of Statement No. 117 are indicated in Chapter 7 of this book.

Recognition Criteria

2.16 *Recognition* is the process of formally reporting an item (asset, liability, revenue, expense, or other element) in the financial statements of an entity. The reported item is depicted in both words and numbers, and the amount is included in the financial statement totals. The disclosure of information by other means (e.g., in notes to financial statements) is *not* recognition. Such disclosure is not a substitute for recognition in financial statements for items that meet recognition criteria.

2.17 An item and information about it should be recognized in financial statements when four fundamental recognition criteria are met:

6 *Financial Statements of Not-for-Profit Organizations* (Norwalk, Connecticut: FASB, 1993).

1. *Definitions*. The item meets the definition of an element of financial statements. (The definitions of elements are provided in Chapter 2 of this book, starting at paragraph 18.)

2. *Measurability*. It has a relevant attribute measurable with sufficient reliability. Five different attributes are used in current practice: historical cost (or proceeds), replacement cost, current market value, net realizable value, and present value of future cash flows. Generally, measurements are stated in nominal units of money, unadjusted for changes in the purchasing power of money over time.

3. *Relevance*. The information about it is capable of making a difference in user decisions.

4. *Reliability*. The information is representationally faithful, verifiable, and neutral.

The four criteria are subject to the pervasive cost/benefit constraint and a materiality threshold.

ELEMENTS OF FINANCIAL STATEMENTS

2.18 SFAC 6 provides definitions for 10 financial statement elements.[7] Seven of these elements (assets, liabilities, equity, revenues, expenses, gains, and losses) appear in the financial statements of both investor-owned and not-for-profit entities. The other three elements (investments by owners, distributions to owners, and comprehensive income) are found only in the financial statements of investor-owned enterprises.

Assets

2.19 Assets are defined in SFAC 6 as "probable future economic benefits obtained or controlled by a particular entity as a result of past transactions or events." The future economic benefit or service potential characteristic of all assets eventually results, directly or indirectly, in future net cash inflows to the entity, whether investor-owned or not-for-profit.

Liabilities

2.20 Liabilities are defined as "probable future sacrifices of economic benefits arising from present obligations of a particular entity to transfer assets or provide services to other entities in the future as a result of past transactions or events."

7 Statement of Financial Accounting Concepts No. 6, "Elements of Financial Statements" (Norwalk, Connecticut: FASB, 1985).

Equity (Net Assets)

2.21 *Equity (net assets)* is defined as "the residual interest in the assets of an entity that remains after deducting its liabilities." The equity of an investor-owned entity differs from that of a not-for-profit organization in that the equity of an investor-owned enterprise may be increased through investments by its owners and decreased by distributions to its owners. (Definitions of investments by owners and distributions to owners are provided in paragraphs 66-67 of SFAC 6.) Not-for-profit hospitals, however, are owned by religious groups, communities, and others who do not invest in and receive ownership returns from these hospitals in the same way as these transactions occur in investor-owned hospitals. There are transfers of ownership interest of not-for-profit organizations and, unlike the implications of the term "not-for-profit," these hospitals must earn a profit in order to maintain capital in a manner similar to investor-owned hospitals. (SFAC No. 6, footnote 10, discusses special ownership characteristics of not-for-profit organizations.)

2.22 The equity of a not-for-profit entity is divided into three mutually exclusive classes:

1. *Permanently Restricted Equity.* This class of equity results from contributed resources whose use by the entity is limited by donor-imposed stipulations that neither expire by passage of time nor can be fulfilled or removed by actions of the entity. The receipt of a perpetual endowment, for example, results in permanently restricted equity.

2. *Temporarily Restricted Equity.* This class of equity results from contributed resources whose use by the entity is limited by donor-imposed stipulations that either expire by passage of time or can be fulfilled and removed by actions of the entity. The receipt of resources whose use is donor-limited to a specific operating purpose (such as for the financing of charity service or medical education and research programs), for example, results in temporarily restricted equity.

3. *Unrestricted Equity.* This class of equity consists of the net assets of the entity that are neither permanently restricted nor temporarily restricted by donor-imposed stipulations. The unrestricted resources of an entity may be used in any manner deemed appropriate by the entity's board of directors and within the broad limits established by the nature and objectives of the entity.

Permanently and temporarily restricted equity relates only to resources restricted by donors. Chart of accounts provisions related to designations made by the hospital board of directors or to limitations imposed by others are discussed in Chapter 5, paragraph 12 of this book.

Revenues

2.23 *Revenues* are defined in SFAC 6 as "inflows or other enhancements of assets of an entity or settlements of its liabilities (or a combination of both) from delivering or producing goods, rendering services, or other activities that constitute the entity's ongoing major and central operations." SFAC 6 also states that revenues represent actual or expected cash inflows that have occurred or will occur as a result of the entity's ongoing major or central operations.

2.24 This definition of revenues has important implications for hospital general-purpose external reporting. It is no longer appropriate to report "gross" revenues (at the hospital's full, established rates) or to report "deductions from gross revenues" arising from charity service, contractual adjustments, and other allowances. Instead, *patient service revenues* are to be reported in the amounts patients or third-party payers have an obligation to pay. The SFAC definition of revenues also means that the term "revenues" should represent actual or anticipated future net cash inflows arising from the hospital's ongoing major or central operations, however that may be defined by the individual hospital. The term "nonoperating revenues" is a contradiction and should not be employed. These matters are discussed in greater detail in Chapter 3.

Expenses

2.25 *Expenses* are defined as "outflows or other using up of assets or incurrences of liabilities (or a combination of both) from delivering or producing goods, rendering services, or carrying out other activities that constitute the entity's ongoing major or central operations." In other words, expenses are actual or anticipated cash outflows (or the equivalent) that have occurred or will occur as a result of an entity's ongoing major or central operations. All expenses, therefore, are operating expenses; the use of the term "nonoperating expenses" should be avoided because it is a contradiction.

Gains

2.26 *Gains* are defined as "increases in equity (net assets) from peripheral or incidental transactions of an entity and other events and circumstances affecting the entity except those that result from revenues or investments by owners." Unlike revenues, gains may be reported as either operating or nonoperating, depending upon the individual entity's definition of its ongoing major or central operations and how the gains relate to that definition.

Losses

2.27 *Losses* are defined as "decreases in equity (net assets) from peripheral or incidental transactions of an entity and from all other transactions and other events and circumstances affecting the entity except those that result from expenses or distributions to owners." Unlike expenses, losses may be reported as either operating or nonoperating, depending upon the individual entity's definition of its ongoing major or central operations and how the losses relate to that definition.

3

Generally Accepted Accounting and Reporting Principles

3.1 Most hospitals issue general-purpose financial statements directed to investors, creditors, other resource providers, and other external users. As discussed in Chapter 2, a complete set of financial statements includes:

- A balance sheet,
- An income statement,
- A statement of changes in equity, and
- A statement of cash flows.

(FASB Statement No. 117, however, does not include an income statement among its requirements for external general-purpose financial reporting by not-for-profit organizations.) The disclosures in accompanying notes and supporting schedules are an integral part of the financial statements. Illustrative financial statements and accompanying notes are provided in Chapter 7.

HIERARCHY OF ACCOUNTING PRINCIPLES

3.2 The financial statements should be prepared in conformity with *generally accepted accounting principles* (GAAP), a technical term that encompasses the conventions, rules, and procedures necessary to define accepted accounting practice at a particular time. These are principles that have substantial authoritative support.

3.3 The most authoritative sources of GAAP for nongovernmental entities are FASB *Statements of Financial Accounting Standards* and *Interpretations*, APB *Opinions*, and the AICPA *Accounting Research Bulletins*. Financial statements issued by governmental hospitals are subject to GASB *Statements* and *Interpretations*, and to FASB and APB pronouncements that the GASB has made specifically applicable to governmental hospitals. (The term "governmental hospital" has not been defined, but a definition is being formulated by GASB.) Accounting issues may arise, however, that are not covered adequately (if at all) by any of these documents, and one must look to other sources for guidance.

3.4 The AICPA Auditing Standards Board identified the sources of established accounting principles that are generally accepted in the United States as follows:[1]

Category

A. Accounting principles promulgated by a body designated by the AICPA Council to establish such principles. (For nongovernmental entities, this is the FASB; for governmental entities, this is the GASB.)

B. Pronouncements of bodies, composed of expert accountants, that deliberate accounting issues in public forums for the purpose of establishing GAAP or describing existing accounting practices that are generally accepted, provided those pronouncements have been exposed for public comment and have been cleared by a body referred to in Category A.

C. Pronouncements of bodies, organized by a body referred to in Category A and composed of expert accountants, that deliberate accounting issues in public forums for the purpose of interpreting or establishing accounting principles or describing existing accounting practices that are generally accepted, or pronouncements referred to in Category B that have been cleared by a body referred to in Category A but have not been exposed for public comment.

D. Practices or pronouncements that are widely recognized as being generally accepted because they represent prevalent practice in a particular industry, or the knowledgeable application to specific circumstances of pronouncements that are generally accepted.

In the absence of sufficient guidance in any of these categories, other accounting literature may be considered. A summary of the hierarchy of generally accepted accounting principles is provided in Figure 3-1. The appropriateness of other accounting literature depends upon its relevance to particular circumstances, the

1 Auditing Standards Board Statement of Auditing Standards No. 69, *The Meaning of Present Fairly in Conformity With Generally Accepted Accounting Principles in the Independent Auditor's Report* (New York: AICPA, 1991).

Figure 3-1
GAAP Hierarchy Summary

Nongovernmental Entities	State and Local Governmental Entities
Established Accounting Principles	
FASB Statements and Interpretations, APB Opinions, and AICPA Accounting Research Bulletins.	GASB Statements and Interpretations, plus any AICPA and FASB pronouncements if made applicable to state and local governments by a GASB Statement or Interpretation.
FASB Technical Bulletins and AICPA Industry Audit and Accounting Guides and AICPA Statements of Position, if cleared by the FASB.	GASB Technical Bulletins, and the following pronouncements if specifically made applicable to state and local governments by the GASB: AICPA Industry Audit and Accounting Guides and AICPA Statements of Position.
Consensus positions of the FASB Emerging Issues Task Force and AICPA Practice Bulletins, if cleared by the FASB.	Consensus positions of a GASB Emerging Issues Task Force (when created) and AICPA Practice Bulletins if specifically made applicable to state and local governments by the GASB.
AICPA accounting interpretations and "Qs and As" published by the FASB staff as well as industry practices widely recognized and prevalent.	"Qs and As" published by the GASB staff, as well as industry practices widely recognized and prevalent.
Other Accounting Literature	
FASB Concepts Statements, APB Statements; AICPA Issues Papers; International Accounting Standards Committee Statements; GASB Statements, Interpretations, and Technical Bulletins; pronouncements of other professional associations or regulatory agencies; AICPA Technical Practice Aids; and accounting textbooks, handbooks, and articles.	GASB Concepts Statements; pronouncements in Categories A through D when not specifically made applicable to state and local governments; APB Statements; FASB Concepts Statements; AICPA Issues Papers; International Accounting Standards Committee Statements; pronouncements of other professional associations or regulatory agencies; AICPA Technical Practice Aids; and accounting textbooks, handbooks, and articles.

specificity of the guidance, and the general recognition of the issuer or author as an authority.

3.5 It is not feasible here to attempt even to summarize all of the pronouncements of the standard-setting bodies. This chapter provides only a brief discussion of selected GAAP related to the particular operating circumstances of hospitals.

THE REPORTING ENTITY AND RELATED ORGANIZATIONS

3.6 The FASB and GASB currently have projects underway that include studies of the *reporting entity concept* and related issues such as the issuance of consolidated or combined financial statements, application of the equity method of accounting for equity investments, and methods of accounting for joint ventures. Current guidelines on these matters are summarized in the following discussion.

3.7 ARB No. 51 addresses the question of whether the financial statements of related or affiliated entities should be consolidated or combined.[2] FAS 94 requires consolidation of majority-owned subsidiary entities except where control is temporary or does not rest with the majority owner.[3] Until new FASB and GASB pronouncements appear, the disclosures required by APB Opinion No. 18 with respect to consolidated and unconsolidated subsidiaries should be made.

3.8 The AICPA has indicated that an entity separate from the hospital is a related organization if one of the two following conditions is met:[4]

1. The hospital controls the separate entity through contracts or other legal documents that give the hospital the authority to direct the separate entity's activities, management, and policies.

2. The hospital is the sole beneficiary of the separate entity. A hospital is the separate entity's sole beneficiary if any one of the three following circumstances exist:

    - The separate entity has solicited resources in the name of the hospital, and with the approval of the hospital, and substantially all of the solicited resources were intended by the contributor to be transferred to the hospital or used at its discretion or direction.

2 Accounting Research Bulletin No. 51, *Consolidated Financial Statements* (New York: AICPA, 1959).

3 Statement of Financial Accounting Standards No. 94, *Consolidation of All Majority-Owned Subsidiaries* (Norwalk, Connecticut: FASB, 1987).

4 *Audits of Providers of Health Care Services* (New York: AICPA), 1990, pp. 127-128.

- The hospital has transferred resources to the separate entity, and substantially all of the separate entity's resources are held for the benefit of the hospital.

- The hospital has assigned certain of its functions (such as the operation of a dormitory) to the separate entity, which is operating primarily for the benefit of the hospital.

3.9 The reporting and disclosure requirements for a hospital having a related organization are summarized in Figure 3-2.[5] Significant relationships and transactions not in the ordinary course of business with directors, management, medical staff, and other related parties should be disclosed in accordance with FAS No. 57.[6]

PATIENT SERVICE REVENUES AND RELATED ISSUES

3.10 Patient service revenues generally are *recorded* on an accrual basis at the hospital's full established rates, regardless of whether or not the hospital expects to collect those amounts. Estimated uncollectible amounts (such as contractual adjustments and charity service) are *recorded* on an accrual basis as *deductions from revenues*. These amounts are subtracted from gross revenues to obtain net revenues for *internal* accounting and managerial purposes.

3.11 In external general-purpose financial statements, however, the *reported* patient service revenue should not include charity service, contractual adjustments, or allowances. Bad debts should be reported as an expense. Thus, the traditional reporting of gross patient service revenues, deductions from revenues, and net patient service revenues is no longer acceptable in these external reports.

3.12 As noted in Chapter 2, paragraph 24, patient service revenue is defined as the amount the patient (or third-party sponsor) has an obligation to pay and will result in cash inflows. Charity services do not result in cash inflows. Cash inflows from third-party payers are defined agreements. Therefore, charity service and contractual adjustments do not qualify for recognition as revenues or receivables in general-purpose financial statements. The same reasoning applies to courtesy discounts granted to employees, clergy, and others.

3.13 The hospital's charity service policy should be disclosed in an appropriate note to the financial statements. This note also should indicate the level of charity service provided in terms of the hospital's charges, costs, units of service, or other

5 *Audits of Providers of Health Care Services* (New York: AICPA, 1990), pp. 127-128.

6 Statement of Financial Accounting Standards No. 57, *Related Party Disclosures* (Norwalk, Connecticut: FASB, 1982).

Figure 3-2
Reporting and Disclosure Requirements for Related Organizations

Circumstances	Requirements
The hospital has a controlling financial interest in another entity as defined in ARB No. 51.*	Issue-consolidated or combined financial statements in accordance with ARB No. 51.
The hospital does not meet the ARB No. 51 criteria, but controls and is the sole beneficiary of the related organization's activities.	In a note to the financial statements, disclose summarized financial data of the related organization (such as total assets, total liabilities, changes in equity, total revenue, total expenses, and amount of distributions to the hospital) and disclose the nature of the relationship between the hospital and the related organization.
Neither of the above is present, but the related organization holds significant amounts of resources designated for the hospital.	Disclose the existence and nature of the relationship and resources held.
There have been material transactions between the hospital and the related organization. (This could be present in any of the foregoing circumstances.)	In notes to the financial statements, disclose the existence and nature of the relationship, and describe and quantify the transactions.

* ARB 51 states that consolidation is necessary when one entity directly or indirectly has a controlling financial interest in another entity. "Controlling financial interest," as a general rule, is evidenced by ownership of more than 50 percent of an organization's voting stock, although it is increasingly recognized that control can exist even though there is less than majority ownership. Other evidences of control, specified in Principles and Practices Board Statement No. 10, include the right to appoint or approve a majority of voting board members, to hire or fire key staff, to approve plans and budgets, or to control debt or plant asset acquisitions.

measurements. (Illustrations of such disclosures appear in P & P Board Statement No. 15.) Disclosures of a similar type also may be made for contractual adjustments.

THIRD-PARTY PAYMENTS

3.14 Under retrospective payment systems, hospitals receive interim payments from third-party payers until a final determination of allowable costs can be made.

In most cases, final settlements will differ from the total of interim payments. Final settlements may not be determined until well after the close of the reporting period. Therefore, it is necessary to record an estimate of the amount receivable from, or payable to, third-party payers so that the receivable or payable is recognized in the same period during which the related services were rendered.

3.15 Another problem arises when certain expenses, gains, or losses enter into the determination of accounting income either before or after they enter into the determination of third-party payment amounts. These timing (temporary) differences are caused by differences between GAAP and the provisions of third-party contracts as to when expenses, gains, or losses are recognized. Timing differences are recognized in the periods in which they *originate* and in the periods in which they *reverse.* P & P Board Statement No. 13 provides accounting guidance on this issue.[7]

3.16 Consider, for example, a payment formula based on an accelerated depreciation method and financial statements based on the straight-line depreciation method. Assuming a depreciable asset having a cost of $45,000 (no salvage value) and an estimated useful life of five years, annual depreciation charges and timing differences would be as follows:

Year	Accelerated Depreciation	SL Depreciation	Timing Differences	
1	$15,000	$9,000	$6,000	Originating
2	12,000	9,000	3,000	Originating
3	9,000	9,000	-0-	
4	6,000	9,000	(3,000)	Reversing
5	3,000	9,000	(6,000)	Reversing
	$45,000	$45,000	$-0-	

Assuming 100% of third-party payments are based on the accelerated depreciation amounts, a timing difference of $6,000 originates in Year 1 and $6,000 of deferred third-party revenue (credit) should be reported in the year-end balance sheet. The balance sheet at the end of Year 2 should report $9,000 of deferred third-party revenue. There is no timing difference originating (or reversing) in Year 3, and the year-end balance sheet continues to report $9,000 of deferred third-party revenue. In Year 4, $3,000 of the accumulated timing difference reverses, and an entry is made to recognize $3,000 of revenue and reduce deferred third-party revenue by

7 Principles and Practices Board Statement No. 13, Timing Differences Pertaining to Third-Party Payment (Westchester, Illinois: HFMA, 1992).

$3,000. The $6,000 remainder of the deferred third-party revenue is recognized as Year 5 revenue.

3.17 This procedure is called *interperiod third-party revenue allocation.* It is employed to achieve a proper matching of recorded expense and earned revenue. Otherwise, for instance, the Year 1 income would include revenue of $15,000 and depreciation expense of only $9,000, resulting in a $6,000 overstatement of Year 1 income.

3.18 In this illustration, the timing differences originating in Years 1 and 2 resulted in a balance sheet deferred *credit.* Other situations may produce a balance sheet deferred *debit.* This will occur when, for example, an expense recognized for accounting purposes in a particular year is greater than the related revenue amount for that year.

3.19 *Permanent differences* arise when, for example, an expense is recognized for accounting purposes but will never be recovered in third-party payments, or a third-party payment is received for which an expense will never be recognized for accounting purposes. Interperiod allocation is not appropriate for permanent differences.

3.20 Changes in third-party payment systems and regulations may affect the recoverability of deferred third-party debits and the realization of deferred third-party credits that have been accumulated because of timing differences. This results in timing difference deferrals becoming permanent differences. In the period when it is determined that the deferred third-party debits and credits in the balance sheet will not be recovered or realized, these amounts should be charged or credited to the income of that period.[8]

INVESTMENTS IN SECURITIES

3.21 Purchased securities initially are recorded at acquisition cost; donated securities are recorded at fair value at date of donation. The hospital's investment in marketable equity securities generally should be reported at market value in conformity with the requirements of FAS 115.[9] Marketable debt securities should be reported at amortized cost if there is the intent and ability to hold these securities until maturity. Otherwise, marketable debt securities generally should be reported at market value. Adjustments to market value generally are reported in a contra-equity account rather than being recognized as charges against or credits to income.

8 Principles and Practices Board Statement No. 13, *Timing Differences Pertaining to Third-Party Payment* (Westchester, Illinois: HFMA, 1992).

9 Statement of Financial Accounting Standards No. 115, *Accounting for Certain Investments in Debt and Equity Securities* (Norwalk, Connecticut: FASB, 1993).

CONTRIBUTIONS RECEIVED

3.22 A contribution is defined as "an unconditional transfer of cash or other assets to an entity, or a settlement or cancellation of its liabilities in a voluntary nonreciprocal transfer by another entity acting other than as an owner."[10] Other assets may include plant assets, securities, services, supplies, and unconditional promises to provide those items in the future.

3.23 Contributions received are measured at their fair values and recognized as revenues or gains, and as assets, in the period received. Not-for-profit hospitals should report donor-restricted contributions received as restricted revenues (support), resulting in an increase in donor-restricted equity. When the donor-imposed restrictions are fulfilled, the amounts of such contributions released from restrictions are reclassified from restricted equity to unrestricted equity. Donor-unrestricted contributions are reported as unrestricted support (revenues or gains) that increases unrestricted equity.

3.24 Contributions received in the form of depreciable assets (or in the form of cash that is donor-restricted to depreciable asset acquisitions) should be reported initially as restricted support. Such contributions are reclassified from donor-restricted equity to unrestricted equity when the depreciable assets are placed in service.

3.25 Contributed resources may be held in trust by another entity that is independent of the hospital. The hospital neither possesses nor controls these resources; they are held and managed by the trustee. When the hospital has no remainder interest in the trust, such resources are not recorded as hospital assets, but appropriate supplementary disclosures are made. If the hospital has a remainder interest, the resources of the trust generally are recorded as hospital assets.

3.26 Distributions from the trust are recorded on the accrual basis as revenues if the distributions are a part of the hospital's ongoing major or central operations, or as gains if the distributions are peripheral and incidental in nature. These distributions should be recorded when the trustee is required to make the distributions. Where the distributions are made at the discretion of the trustee, the hospital records the distributions according to the terms of the trust document or the agreement with the trustee. Supplementary disclosure should be made of the hospital's right to future income and the principal amount held in the trust.

3.27 Unrestricted grants, tax support, and subsidies received from governmental or community agencies should be reported as revenues or as gains, depending upon whether they are a part of the hospital's ongoing major or central operations or are peripheral and incidental in nature.

10 Statement of Financial Accounting Standards No. 116, *Accounting for Contributions Received and Contributions Made* (Norwalk, Connecticut: FASB, 1993), p.2.

3.28 Contributed services usually are not recorded. If all of the following criteria are met, however, the fair value of such services is given accounting recognition:

- The services received create or enhance nonfinancial assets or require specialized skills.
- The services received are provided by individuals possessing specialized skills.
- The services received generally would be purchased by the hospital if not provided by donation.
- The dollar value of the services is reasonably measurable.

If donated services meet these criteria, they are usually related to the hospital's ongoing major or central activities and are recorded as revenue and expense.

THE THREE-PART EQUITY CONCEPT

3.29 The equity (net assets) of a hospital is the difference between total assets and total liabilities. Equity is increased by revenues and gains, and is decreased by expenses and losses. An investor-owned hospital's equity also is increased by investments of assets by its owners, and is decreased by distributions of assets to its owners. In contrast, not-for-profit hospitals are owned by religious groups, communities, and others who do not invest in and receive ownership returns in the same way as these transactions occur in investor-owned hospitals. The not-for-profit hospital's equity is increased by income from its operating activities and by receipt of assets from donors who impose temporary or permanent restrictions on the use of those assets.

3.30 The equity accounts of an investor-owned hospital are largely the same as those of other investor-owned entities, but the equity accounts of a not-for-profit hospital are considerably different. These differences result from the receipt of donor-restricted resources. Donors contribute resources to the hospital to permit it to maintain or increase its capacity to provide services. The receipt of donated resources increases the assets of the hospital, and also imposes a fiduciary responsibility on its management to use the assets effectively. That responsibility, however, generally does not constitute a liability (as defined in Chapter 2, paragraph 20). It differs from the responsibility imposed by incurring a liability, which involves a creditor's claim.

3.31 The receipt of unrestricted donated assets generally is recorded as an increase in unrestricted assets and in revenues or gains (depending upon the hospital's ongoing major or central operations). The receipt of donor-restricted assets generally is recorded as an increase in assets and in restricted equity. Subsequently, when the donor's stipulations either expire by passage of time or are fulfilled or otherwise removed, the recorded amount of those assets is reclassified from donor-restricted equity to unrestricted equity. These reclassifications are reported in the statement of income and other changes in unrestricted equity as shown in Chapter 7.

3.32 This means that the equity of a not-for-profit hospital (whether or not a fund accounting system is employed) should be divided into three primary, and mutually exclusive, classes: unrestricted equity, temporarily donor-restricted equity, and permanently donor-restricted equity. These three classes of equity are described in Chapter 5, paragraph 37.

FUND ACCOUNTING AND REPORTING

3.33 Many hospitals receive significant amounts of resources from donors and grantors who impose restrictions on the use of the donated resources. A fiduciary responsibility arises to comply with donors' restrictions, and some hospitals employ a *fund accounting* system to meet that responsibility. Fund accounting also is used by governmental hospitals to help assure compliance with legislative restrictions.

3.34 In a fund accounting system, the hospital's assets (and related liabilities and equity) are segregated into self-balancing sets of accounts (called *funds*) that are established and maintained to account for specific activities and the attainment of certain objectives in accordance with legal and other externally imposed restrictions. Each fund is viewed as a separate and distinct fiscal and accounting entity.

3.35 Some hospitals use fund accounting techniques only for internal accounting and managerial control purposes. In external reporting, the fund classifications are not used; the assets and liabilities of all funds are presented in an *aggregated* (or *single fund*) format as illustrated in Chapter 7. While hospitals may report their assets and liabilities by fund (in a disaggregated format), this practice is not encouraged by the FASB and other authoritative bodies.

3.36 HFMA Principles and Practices Board (PPB) Statement Number 8, *The Use of Fund Accounting and the Need for Single Fund Reporting by Institutional Healthcare Providers,* takes the position that general-purpose financial statements of hospitals should be comparable to the reporting of other businesses.[11] In other words, assets, liabilities, and equity should be presented in a single aggregated balance sheet without differentiation by fund. The PPB concluded that this form of presentation (single fund reporting) should be used by all hospitals, but the use of a fund accounting system for internal managerial purposes is a matter to be decided by the individual hospital.

11 *A Compilation of Statements 1-8* (Westchester, Illinois: HFMA, 1987), p. 63.

Unrestricted (General) Fund

3.37 In fund accounting, the unrestricted fund (often referred to as the general fund) is used to account for hospital assets (as well as the related liabilities) that are not donor-restricted to particular uses. Plant assets, and the related long-term debt, are recorded in the unrestricted fund. In addition, all unrestricted revenues, expenses, gains, and losses are recorded in the unrestricted fund.

3.38 In addition, the unrestricted fund includes assets whose use is designated or limited by parties other than donors:

- Assets designated by the governing board for certain purposes, e.g., assets board-designated for capital expenditures. The board, however, has the power to rescind its designations and use the resources for other purposes.
- Assets (sometimes held by trustees) whose use is limited in accordance with the terms of bond indentures or contractual agreements with external parties other than donors.

That portion of these assets required to meet current liabilities should be reported among the hospital's current assets as shown in Figure 7-1.

3.39 A hospital may have possession of assets owned by others under an agency relationship. These assets are included in the unrestricted fund. A liability is recorded upon receipt of such assets. When the assets are disbursed or returned, the liability is eliminated. Accounting for agency funds is discussed in P & P Board Statement No. 5.

Restricted Funds

3.40 There is one, and only one, unrestricted fund, but hospitals may maintain several different types of funds to account for resources that are temporarily or permanently donor-restricted:

1. Temporarily donor-restricted funds—
   - Specific-Purpose Funds,
   - Plant Replacement and Expansion Funds, and
   - Term Endowment Funds.
2. Permanently donor-restricted funds—
   - Permanent Endowment Funds.

It may be necessary to maintain two or more funds of each type, e.g., a hospital may need to maintain a number of different specific purpose funds. Although a separate accounting may be required, donor-restricted funds generally can be grouped in the major categories indicated.

3.41 *Specific-Purpose Funds* are used to account for resources that are temporarily restricted by donors for the support of educational programs, research projects, charity services, and other specific operating activities (excluding acquisition of plant assets). Receipts of such resources are initially recorded as restricted revenues of the specific-purpose fund, resulting in increases in temporarily donor-restricted equity. In the period during which expenditures are required for the donor-specified purposes or when the time specified by the donor has elapsed, these amounts are reclassified from restricted equity to unrestricted equity, being reported as "assets released from donor restrictions." Income from investments of a specific purpose fund generally is recorded as an addition to restricted equity. If this income is not donor-restricted, however, the income is properly recorded in the unrestricted fund. Gains (losses) on sales of these investments usually are recorded as additions to (reductions of) restricted equity.

3.42 *Plant Replacement and Expansion Funds* are used to account for those resources that are temporarily donor-restricted for plant asset acquisition and capital debt retirement. (This donor-restricted fund should not be used to record plant assets or funded depreciation amounts.) Receipts of these donor-restricted resources are recorded as restricted revenues and increases in temporarily donor-restricted equity. In the periods in which the donor-imposed restrictions are fulfilled, these amounts are reclassified from restricted equity to unrestricted equity, being reported as "assets released from donor restrictions" as illustrated in Chapter 7.

Income from investments of plant replacement and expansion funds usually is recorded as an addition to restricted equity. If this income is not donor-restricted, however, it is recorded in the unrestricted fund and is reported as unrestricted revenues or gains. Gains (losses) on sales of these investments usually are recorded as additions to (reductions of) restricted equity.

3.43 *Term Endowment Funds* are maintained to account for resources that are temporarily donor-restricted to investments. If the donor specifies how the investment income must be used, the income is recorded in the appropriate restricted fund as an addition to equity. When the donor does not specify how the investment income may be used, the income is recorded in the unrestricted fund as unrestricted revenues or gains. Upon expiration of a term endowment, the principal amount is reclassified from the term endowment fund equity to the equity of another restricted fund or to unrestricted revenues (or gains), depending upon the donor's stipulations.

3.44 *Permanent Endowment Funds* are similar to term endowment funds except that the resources are permanently donor-restricted to investments; the restriction is perpetual and does not expire. Investment income is recorded in the unrestricted fund or in an appropriate restricted fund, depending upon the donor's stipulations. Gains (losses) arising from sales of investments of permanent endowment funds generally are credited (charged) directly to the permanent endowment fund balance.

FINANCIAL STATEMENTS

3.45 A relatively recent development in general-purpose financial reporting is the presentation of a Statement of Cash Flows (instead of a Statement of Changes in Financial Position) as prescribed in FAS No. 95.[12] A similar statement is required by GASB for governmental hospitals.[13] Chapter 7 provides illustrations and further discussion of the Statement of Cash Flows as well as other hospital financial statements. Particular attention is given to the financial statement formats described in FAS No. 115.[14]

12 Statement of Financial Accounting Standards No. 95, *Statement of Cash Flows* (Norwalk, Connecticut: FASB, 1987). Although FAS 95 specifically excludes not-for-profit hospitals from its scope, the AICPA has indicated that not-for-profit hospitals should apply the provisions of FAS 95 to ensure that their statements of cash flows are comparable with those of investor-owned entities.

13 GASB Statement No. 9, *Reporting Cash Flows of Proprietary and Nonexpendable Trust Funds and Governmental Entities That Use Proprietary Fund Accounting* (Norwalk, Connecticut: GASB, 1989).

14 *Financial Statements of Not-for-Profit Organizations* (Norwalk, Connecticut: FASB, 1993).

4

Overview of the Chart of Accounts

4.1 A chart of accounts is a list of account titles (with numerical coding) designed for the compilation of financial data concerning the assets, liabilities, equity, revenues, expenses, gains, and losses of an enterprise. It should provide for an accumulation of information in a manner that is as useful as possible for managerial planning and control purposes. This requires that the classification of revenues and expenses in the chart of accounts should correspond to the division of authority and responsibility in the hospital as depicted by its organization chart. A system of *responsibility accounting and reporting* should be employed so that (1) expenses are classified according to the organizational units incurring them and (2) revenues are classified according to the organizational units in which they are earned.

4.2 Although the chart of accounts is designed primarily to meet the informational needs of hospital management, the requirements of investors, creditors, third-party payers, donors, taxing and regulatory agencies, oversight bodies, and other external parties also influence its design.

4.3 Because no two hospitals are, or should be, organized in precisely the same manner, no two hospitals will employ identical charts of accounts. It therefore is not possible to develop a chart of accounts that will meet all of the requirements of all hospitals. For this reason, no attempt is made in this book to provide an exhaustive list of accounts. The chart of accounts (including the numerical coding system) described here is illustrative and representative. The nature and use of these accounts are discussed in Chapters 5 and 6.

4.4 Some hospitals may not require all of the detailed information provided by the illustrative chart of accounts; other hospitals may need even more detailed information. A fairly wide range of accounts is included here because it usually is easier for the individual hospital to omit that which is not required than to add what is required but not described in this manual. The illustrative chart of accounts can be contracted or expanded to meet specific hospital requirements without significantly affecting the basic consistency necessary for external financial reporting purposes.

NUMERICAL CODING SYSTEM

4.5 The numerical coding system described in this illustrative chart of accounts consists of 11 digits divided into five fields:

00-00-0-0000-00

Field 1: Entity Designator

Field 2: Fund Designator

Field 3: Financial Statement Element

Field 4: Primary Subclassification

Field 5: Secondary Subclassification

Field 1: Entity Designator

4.6 The primary prefix of two digits is the *entity designator:*

Primary Prefix		
01	Parent Organization	01-00-0-0000-00
02	Hospital "A"	02-00-0-0000-00
03	Hospital "B"	03-00-0-0000-00
04	Hospital "C"	04-00-0-0000-00
05	Skilled Nursing Facility	05-00-0-0000-00
Etc.		

If, for example, a hospital is one of two or more subsidiary entities controlled by a parent organization, the primary prefix is employed to separately identify the accounts of the parent organization and of each subsidiary. This facilitates the preparation of consolidated or combined financial statements for the affiliated group of entities. *Hospitals that are not a component of an affiliated group of entities will not use this primary prefix in their numerical coding systems.*

Field 2: Fund Designator

4.7 The secondary prefix of two digits is the *fund designator* for hospitals whose accounting records are maintained under a fund accounting system:

Secondary Prefix		
10	Unrestricted (General) Fund	00-10-0-0000-00
	Temporarily Donor-Restricted Funds -	
20	Specific-Purpose Funds	00-20-0-0000-00
30	Plant Replacement and Expansion Funds	00-30-0-0000-00
40	Term Endowment Funds	00-40-0-0000-00
	Permanently Donor-Restricted Funds -	
50	Permanent Endowment Funds	00-50-0-0000-00
Etc.		

The fundamentals of fund accounting are discussed in Chapter 3, starting at paragraph 3.33. *Hospitals that do not employ a fund accounting system will not use this secondary prefix in their numerical coding systems.*

Field 3: Financial Statement Element

4.8 The single-digit field designates the *basic financial statement element* within which each of the accounts in the hospital's chart of accounts is properly included. Digits 1, 2, and 3 specify balance sheet accounts, as well as accounts that appear in a statement of changes in equity (or a statement of changes in fund balances, where fund accounting is employed); digits 4 through 9 are used to identify accounts that are included in a statement of income and other changes in unrestricted equity.

Digit	Balance Sheet and Statement of Changes in Equity	
1	Assets	00-00-1-0000-00
2	Liabilities	00-00-2-0000-00
3	Equity (Net Assets)	00-00-3-0000-00

Digit	Statement of Income and Other Changes in Unrestrcted Equity	
4	Revenues—Patient Services	00-00-4-0000-00
5	Deductions from Revenues; Other Revenues; Assets Released from Donor Restrictions	00-00-5-0000-00
6	Expenses—Patient Services	00-00-6-0000-00
7	Expenses—General, Fiscal, and Administrative Services	00-00-7-0000-00
8	Expenses—Research and Education; Unassigned Expenses	00-00-8-0000-00
9	Nonoperating Gains and Losses	00-00-9-0000-00

As discussed in Chapter 2, paragraph 23, the amount to be reported as revenues is the amount the hospital expects to collect. This means that "Deductions from Revenues" (such as contractual adjustments and charity service) are not included as a basic element in the body of statements of income and other changes in equity issued for external reporting purposes. Such "deductions," however, are appropriately disclosed in the notes accompanying the financial statements. Hospitals probably will need to continue to record revenues at established rates, as well as the related revenue deductions, and include those amounts in reports prepared for internal purposes. It is only for this reason that the illustrative chart includes accounts for revenue deductions.

Field 4: Primary Subclassification

4.9 The four-digit field provides for a subclassification of the fundamental financial statement elements into the primary accounts used by the hospital. The manner in which the four digits in this field may be employed is illustrated in subsequent sections of this chapter. Should four digits not meet the needs of the individual hospital, this field may be expanded to five digits (or contracted to three digits).

Field 5: Secondary Subclassification

4.10 The two-digit suffix provides for a secondary detailed classification of the primary accounts. The manner in which this suffix is used for balance sheet accounts depends upon the particular requirements of the individual hospital. A discussion and illustration of the use of the suffix for revenue and expense accounts is provided at a later point in this chapter, starting at paragraph 16. Should a two-digit suffix be inadequate, the suffix may be increased to three or more digits to accommodate more detailed informational needs.

BALANCE SHEET AND STATEMENT OF CHANGES IN EQUITY ACCOUNTS

4.11 The basic elements of balance sheets are designated by the single-digit field, using the numerals 1, 2, or 3:

Single-Digit Field		
1	Assets	00-00-1-000-00
2	Liabilities	00-00-2-000-00
3	Equity (Net Assets)	00-00-3-000-00

Equity accounts also include those that are presented in statements of changes in equity (or statements of changes in fund balances, when fund accounting is employed).

4.12 These three basic elements of the balance sheet are further classified by the use of numerals in the four-digit field. The *first* digit in this field is used to designate the following:

First Digit	ASSETS	
1	Cash	00-00-1-1000-00
2	Short-Term Investments	00-00-1-2000-00
3	Receivables—Patients	00-00-1-3000-00
4	Other Receivables	00-00-1-4000-00
5	Other Current Assets	00-00-1-5000-00
6	Long-Term Investments	00-00-1-6000-00
7	Assets Whose Use Is Limited or Restricted	00-00-1-7000-00
8	Property, Plant, and Equipment	00-00-1-8000-00
9	Other Noncurrent Assets	00-00-1-9000-00
	LIABILITIES	
1	Current Portion of Long-Term Debt	00-00-2-1000-00
2	Short-Term Notes and Loans Payable	00-00-2-2000-00
3	Accounts Payable	00-00-2-3000-00
4	Accrued Employee Compensation and Related Liabilities	00-00-2-4000-00
5	Other Accrued Expenses	00-00-2-5000-00
6	Deferred Credits	00-00-2-6000-00

First Digit	LIABILITIES (continued)	
7	Other Current Liabilities	00-00-2-7000-00
8	Long-Term Debt	00-00-2-8000-00
9	Other Noncurrent Liabilities	00-00-2-9000-00
	EQUITY	
	Not-for-Profit Hospitals	
1	Equity—Unrestricted	00-00-3-1000-00
	Equity—Temporarily Donor-Restricted:	
2	For Specific Operating Purposes	00-00-3-2000-00
3	For Plant Replacement and Expansion	00-00-3-3000-00
4	For Term Endowments	00-00-3-4000-00
5	Equity—Permanently Donor-Restricted	00-00-3-5000-00
6	Investor-Owned Hospital Corporations	00-00-3-6000-00
7	Investor-Owned Hospital Partnerships	00-00-3-7000-00
Etc.		

4.13 The *second, third,* and *fourth* digits in the four-digit field for balance sheet accounts are used to provide a more specific identification of the primary asset, liability, and equity accounts. Any account in the "1-1000" series, for example, is a cash account. A general checking account may be numbered "1-1100," a payroll checking account may be numbered "1-1200," and so on. The manner in which the four-digit field may be used to designate the primary balance sheet accounts is indicated in the following section of this chapter. The two-digit suffix to the balance sheet account numbers may be employed to obtain a secondary subclassification of the accounts according to the requirements of the individual hospital.

4.14 Figure 4-1 presents an illustrative outline of the primary balance sheet and statement of changes in equity accounts that may be employed by a hospital. The indicated account numbers do not include either the primary prefix (entity designator) or the secondary prefix (fund designator). A discussion of these accounts appears in Chapter 5.

Figure 4-1
Outline of Balance Sheet Accounts

Account Numbers	Account Titles
	CURRENT ASSETS
1-1000-00	**Cash**
1-1100-00	General Checking Accounts
1-1200-00	Payroll Checking Accounts
1-1300-00	Other Checking Accounts
1-1400-00	Imprest Cash Funds
1-1500-00	Savings Accounts
1-1600-00	Certificates of Deposit
1-1700-00	U.S. Treasury Bills and Notes
1-1900-00	Assets Whose Use Is Limited and Required for Current Liabilities
1-2000-00	**Short-Term Investments**
1-2100-00	Government Securities
1-2200-00	Corporate Bonds
1-2300-00	Corporate Stocks
1-3000-00	**Receivables—Patient-Specific**
1-3100-00	Inpatient Receivables
1-3110-00	In-house
1-3120-00	Discharged—Unbilled
1-3130-00	Discharged—Billed—Medicare Standard Arrangement
1-3140-00	Discharged—Billed—Public Aid Programs
1-3150-00	Discharged—Billed—Charge-Based Third Parties
1-3160-00	Discharged—Billed—Third-Party Risk Arrangements
1-3170-00	Discharged—Billed—Other Third Parties
1-3180-00	Discharged—Billed—Self-Pay
1-3200-00	Outpatient Receivables
1-3220-00	Unbilled
1-3230-00	Billed—Medicare Standard Arrangement
1-3240-00	Billed—Public Aid Programs
1-3250-00	Billed—Charge-Based Third Parties
1-3260-00	Billed—Third-Party Risk Arrangements
1-3270-00	Billed—Other Third Parties
1-3280-00	Billed—Self-Pay

Account Numbers	Account Titles
	CURRENT ASSETS
1-3300-00	Allowance for Uncollectible Receivables
1-3310-00	Bad Debts
1-3320-00	Contractual Adjustments
1-3330-00	Charity Service
1-3340-00	Courtesy Discounts
1-3350-00	Other
1-4000-00	**Other Receivables**
1-4100-00	Due from Third-Party Payers
1-4200-00	Pledges Receivable
1-4250-00	Allowance for Uncollectible Pledges
1-4300-00	Grants and Legacies Receivable
1-4400-00	Due from Staff and Employees
1-4500-00	Due from Affiliated Organizations
1-4600-00	Due from Other Funds
1-4700-00	Accrued Interest Receivable
1-4800-00	Dividends Receivable
1-5000-00	**Other Current Assets**
1-5100-00	Inventory
1-5110-00	General Stores
1-5120-00	Pharmacy
1-5130-00	Central Supply
1-5140-00	Dietary
1-5150-00	Plant Operation and Maintenance
1-5200-00	Prepaid Expenses
1-5210-00	Insurance
1-5220-00	Interest
1-5230-00	Rent
1-5240-00	Pension Plan Expense
1-5300-00	Deferred Income Taxes
1-5400-00	Deferred Third-Party Debits

Account Numbers	Account Titles
	NONCURRENT ASSETS
1-6000-00	**Long-Term Investments**
1-6100-00	Government Securities
1-6200-00	Corporate Bonds
1-6300-00	Corporate Stocks
1-6400-00	Investments in Affiliated Entities
1-7000-00	**Assets Whose Use Is Limited or Restricted**
1-7100-00	By Board for Capital Improvements
1-7200-00	By Third-Party Payers for Funded Depreciation
1-7300-00	By Malpractice Funding Arrangement - Held by Trustee
1-7400-00	By Bond Indenture - Held by Trustee
1-7500-00	By Donors for Specific Purposes
1-7600-00	By Donors for Plant Replacement and Expansion Purposes
1-7700-00	By Donors for Term Endowment Purposes
1-7800-00	By Donors for Permanent Endowment Purposes
1-7900-00	Assets Whose Use Is Limited or Restricted Reclassified to Current Assets
1-8000-00	**Property, Plant, and Equipment**
1-8100-00	Land
1-8200-00	Land Improvements
1-8300-00	Buildings
1-8400-00	Leasehold Improvements
1-8500-00	Fixed Equipment
1-8600-00	Major Movable Equipment
1-8700-00	Minor Equipment
1-8800-00	Construction in Progress
1-8900-00	Accumulated Depreciation
1-8982-00	Land Improvements
1-8983-00	Buildings
1-8984-00	Leasehold Improvements
1-8985-00	Fixed Equipment
1-8986-00	Major Movable Equipment

Account Numbers	Account Titles
	NONCURRENT ASSETS (continued)
1-9000-00	**Other Noncurrent Assets**
1-9100-00	Nonoperating Plant Assets
1-9200-00	Accumulated Depreciation - Nonoperating Plant Assets
1-9300-00	Deferred Financing Costs
1-9400-00	Intangible Assets
1-9410-00	Goodwill
1-9420-00	Other
1-9500-00	Deferred Income Taxes
1-9600-00	Deferred Third-Party Debits
	CURRENT LIABILITIES
2-1000-00	**Current Maturities of Long-Term Debt**
2-2000-00	**Short-Term Notes and Loans Payable**
2-2100-00	Banks
2-2200-00	Vendors
2-2300-00	Others
2-3000-00	**Accounts Payable**
2-3100-00	Trade Accounts
2-3200-00	Other Accounts
2-4000-00	**Accrued Employee Compensation and Related Liabilities**
2-4100-00	Accrued Payroll
2-4200-00	Accrued Vacation, Holiday, and Sick Pay
2-4300-00	Taxes Withheld and Accrued
2-4310-00	Income Taxes
2-4320-00	Social Security Taxes
2-4400-00	Unemployment Taxes Payable
2-4500-00	Accrued Workmens' Compensation Insurance Premiums
2-4600-00	Accrued Hospitalization Insurance Premiums
2-4700-00	Union Dues Payable
2-4800-00	Accrued Pension Plan Liability
2-4900-00	Obligation for Other Postemployment Benefits

Account Numbers	Account Titles
	CURRENT LIABILITIES (continued)
2-5000-00	**Other Accrued Expenses Payable**
2-5100-00	Interest
2-5200-00	Rent
2-5300-00	Property Taxes
2-5400-00	Fees Payable to Medical Specialists
2-5500-00	Current Portion of Estimated Malpractice Costs
2-6000-00	**Deferred Credits**
2-6100-00	Deferred Income
2-6200-00	Deferred Income Taxes
2-6300-00	Deferred Third-Party Revenue
2-6400-00	Patients' Deposits
2-6500-00	Unidentified Receipts
2-6600-00	Patients' Credit Balances
2-7000-00	**Other Current Liabilities**
2-7100-00	Advances from Third-Party Payers
2-7200-00	Due to Third-Party Payers
2-7300-00	Dividends Payable
2-7400-00	Income Taxes Payable
2-7500-00	Due to Affiliated Entities
2-7600-00	Due to Other Funds
2-7700-00	Construction Contracts Payable
	NONCURRENT LIABILITIES
2-8000-00	**Long-Term Debt**
2-8100-00	Mortgages Payable
2-8200-00	Notes Payable
2-8300-00	Bonds Payable
2-8310-00	Term Bonds Payable
2-8320-00	Serial Bonds Payable
2-8380-00	Unamortized Bond Premium
2-8390-00	Unamortized Bond Discount

Account Numbers	Account Titles
	NONCURRENT LIABILITIES
2-8400-00	Obligation Under Capital Leases
2-8500-00	Pension Plan Liability
2-8600-00	Other Postretirement Benefits Liability
2-9000-00	**Other Noncurrent Liabilities**
2-9100-00	Deferred Credits
2-9110-00	Deferred Income
2-9120-00	Deferred Income Taxes
2-9130-00	Deferred Third-Party Revenue
2-9200-00	Estimated Malpractice Costs
	EQUITY
	Not-for-Profit Hospitals
3-1000-00	**Equity—Unrestricted**
3-1100-00	Income Summary
3-1200-00	Interequity Reclassifications
3-1300-00	Prior Period Adjustments
	Equity—Temporarily Donor-Restricted
3-2000-00	**For Specific Operating Purposes**
3-2100-00	Donated Resources Received
3-2200-00	Investment Income
3-2300-00	Interequity Reclassifications
3-3000-00	**For Plant Replacement and Expansion**
3-3100-00	Donated Resources Received
3-3200-00	Investment Income
3-3300-00	Interequity Reclassifications
3-4000-00	**For Term Endowments**
3-4100-00	Donated Resources Received
3-4200-00	Investment Gains and Losses
3-4300-00	Interequity Reclassifications
3-5000-00	**Equity—Permanently Donor-Restricted**
3-5100-00	Donated Resources Received
3-5200-00	Investment Gains and Losses

Account Numbers	Account Titles
	EQUITY
	Investor-Owned Hospital Corporations
3-6000-00	**Stockholders' Equity**
3-6100-00	Capital Stock
3-6200-00	Additional Contributed Capital
3-6300-00	Retained Earnings
3-6310-00	Prior Period Adjustments
3-6320-00	Income Summary
3-6330-00	Dividends Paid
3-6400-00	Treasury Stock
	Investor-Owned Hospital Partnership
3-7000-00	Partners' Equity
3-7100-00	Income Summary
3-7200-00	Partners' Drawings

STATEMENT OF INCOME AND OTHER CHANGES IN UNRESTRICTED EQUITY ACCOUNTS

4.15 As noted earlier, the basic elements of statement of income and other changes in unrestricted equity are designated by the single-digit field, using the numerals 4 through 9:

Single-Digit Field		
1, 2, 3	(Balance Sheet and Statement of Changes in Equity Accounts)	
4	Revenues—Patient Services	00-00-4-0000-00
5	Deductions from Revenues; Other Revenues; Assets Released from Donor Restrictions	00-00-5-0000-00
6	Expenses—Patient Services	00-00-6-0000-00
7	Expenses—General, Fiscal, and Administrative Services	00-00-7-0000-00
8	Expenses—Research and Education, Unassigned Expenses	00-00-8-0000-00
9	Nonoperating Gains and Losses	00-00-9-0000-00

Designation of the Four-Digit Field and the Two-Digit Suffix

4.16 For most revenue and expense accounts, the four-digit field will designate revenue and expense responsibility centers in a manner that conforms to the hospital's organizational structure. The most likely uses of the two-digit suffix are as follows:

- The two-digit suffix to patient service revenue accounts should be used to provide a classification of those revenues by type of patient (inpatient or outpatient) and by type of payor (payment source) as illustrated in Figure 4-2. The use of the two-digit suffix for other revenue (and gain) accounts will depend upon the particular informational requirements of the individual hospital.
- The two-digit suffix to expense accounts (other than those in the unassigned expense category) should be used to provide a natural (object of expenditure) classification as suggested in Figure 4-3. The use of the two-digit suffix for other expense (and loss) accounts will depend upon the particular informational requirements of the individual hospital.

4.17 In addition, the hospital may choose to expand the two-digit suffix to three or more digits if two digits prove to be inadequate. A number of different types of revenue and expense subsidiary records also can be maintained to provide additional details relating to certain kinds of revenues and expenses. For example, an insurance register might be employed to supply detailed subsidiary information concerning insurance expense; a plant and equipment subsidiary ledger record can be used to provide detailed information about depreciation expense.

Figure 4-2
Use of the Two-Digit Suffix
Patient Service Revenue Accounts

First Digit	Type of Patient
1	Inpatient
2	Outpatient

Second Digit	Type of Payor (Payment Source)*
1	Medicare Standard Arrangement
2	Public Aid Programs
3	Charge-Based Third Parties
4	Third-Party Risk Arrangements
5	Other Third Parties
6	Self-Pay

*Defined in Chapter 5, paragraph 5.

Figure 4-3
Use of Two-Digit Suffix
Natural Classification of Expenses

Two-Digit Suffix

00 **Salaries and Wages**

Salaries and wages are defined as (1) all remuneration, payable in cash, for services performed by employees for the hospital, and (2) the fair market value of services donated to the hospital by persons meeting the criteria described in Chapter 3, paragraph 28. Payments to independent contractors such as private-duty nurses should be excluded.

01 Management and Supervision

Employees included in this classification of salaries and wages are primarily involved in the direction, supervision, and coordination of hospital activities. This includes employees having job titles such as president, chief executive officer, chief fiscal officer, vice president, manager, director, department head, and supervisor. These employees are exempt from federal wage and hour laws.

02 Technicians and Specialists

Employees included in this classification of salaries and wages usually perform activities of a creative or complex nature. This includes employees having job titles such as therapist, technologist, technician, programmer, instructor, coordinator, accountant, chef, plumber, and carpenter. In many cases, these employees are licensed or registered. Some of these positions are exempt from federal wage and hour laws.

03 Registered Nurses

This classification includes only registered nurses who provide direct nursing care to patients. Registered nurses performing supervisory functions should be classified as Management and Supervision (01). Registered nurses who function as instructors or coordinators should be classified as Technicians and Specialists (02).

04 Licensed Vocational (Practical) Nurses

This classification includes licensed vocational (practical) nurses who provide direct nursing care to patients. Those not providing direct patient care should be classified as Technicians and Specialists (02). Employees in this classification (04) are subject to federal wage and hour laws.

05 Aides and Orderlies

Included in this classification are nontechnical personnel who provide direct nursing care to patients. These employees have job titles such as aide, orderly, and nurse assistant, and they are subject to federal wage and hour laws.

06 Clerical and Other Administrative Employees

Included in this classification are nontechnical personnel who perform record keeping, communication, and other administrative functions, and they are subject to federal wage and hour laws. Examples of job titles are accounting clerk, messenger, secretary, telephone operator, clerk-typist, cashier, and receptionist.

07 Environment and Food Service Employees

This classification includes personnel who provide basic services related to food and accommodations. They perform routine work of a nontechnical nature, and are subject to federal wage and hour laws. Examples of job titles are maintenance worker, housekeeping aide, cook's helper, flatwork finisher, guard, food service worker, wall washer, and washperson.

08 Physicians

Employees included in this classification are employed for consulting, diagnosing, and prescribing and providing treatment for patients. These personnel must possess doctor of medicine or doctor of osteopathy degrees and be licensed to practice medicine.

09 Nonphysician Medical Practitioners

Employees included in this classification are employed for consulting, diagnosing, and prescribing and providing treatment to patients under the direction of a physician. Job titles include nurse practitioner, physician's assistant, and clinical specialist.

10 Vacation, Holiday, Sick Pay, and Other Nonworked Compensation

This classification should be charged with all compensation for time not worked. Included are vacation pay, holiday pay, sick pay, military leave, funerals, and education. (Time allowed and paid for coffee breaks, lunch breaks, and in-service education is considered to be worked time.)

15 Employee Benefits

Responsibility center managers have little or no control over most employee benefits. Because of this, many hospitals do not charge employees benefits directly to responsibility center expense accounts as a part of the regular accounting routine. Instead, the costs of such benefits are charged to unassigned expense account 8-7500 (Employee Benefits).

Other hospitals, however, choose to charge the costs of such benefits to responsibility center accounts as direct expenses. Where this is done, the two-digit suffix may be used as follows:

16 Social Security Taxes

17 State and Federal Unemployment Taxes

18 Group Health and Life Insurance

19 Retirement Plan Expense

20 Workmen's Compensation Insurance

21 Group Disability Insurance

25 **Professional Fees—Medical**

26 Physicians' Remuneration

This classification should include all fees paid to nonemployee physicians for patient care and supervisory activities.

27 Therapists and Others (Nonphysician)

This classification should include all fees paid to therapists and others (nonphysician) for patient care.

30 **Other Professional Fees**

31 Consulting and Management Services

32 Legal Services

33 Auditing Services

40 Departmental Supplies and Materials

The two-digit suffix 40 through 44 may be used to record the costs of specialized departmental supplies and materials that are unique and are indigenous to a particular department. Some examples are food in Dietary, film in Radiology, and reagents in the Laboratory.

45 **General Supplies and Materials**

General supplies and materials are those that are common to many departments. The costs of these supplies and materials may be subclassified as indicated below:

46 Office and Administrative Supplies

47 Employee Wearing Apparel

48 Instruments and Minor Medical Equipment (Nondepreciable)

49 Minor Equipment (Nondepreciable)

50 Other Supplies and Materials

60 **Purchased Services**

The two-digit suffix 60 through 74 may be used to record the costs of purchased services as indicated below:

61 Medical—Purchased Services

62 Repairs and Maintenance—Purchased Services

63 Medical School Contracts—Purchased Services

64 Management Services

65 Collection Services

66 Utilities

67 Telephone

68 Dues and Subscriptions

69 Travel

75 **Other Direct Expenses**

80 **Depreciation and Other Indirect Expenses**

Many hospitals do not charge expenses such as depreciation, rentals, insurance, licenses, and taxes directly to the responsibility centers. Instead, they are charged to the appropriate accounts in the unassigned expenses classification.

Other hospitals charge all or some of these expenses to the responsibility centers as a part of the regular accounting routine. Where this procedure is followed, the two-digit suffix 80 through 99 may be employed as indicated below:

81 Depreciation—Land Improvements

82 Depreciation—Buildings

83 Depreciation—Leasehold Improvements

84 Depreciation—Fixed Equipment

85 Depreciation—Major Movable Equipment

86 Rentals—Land

87 Rentals—Buildings

88 Rentals—Equipment

90 Insurance

95 Licenses

96 Taxes—Property

97 Taxes—Income

98 Taxes—Other

Linking the Chart of Accounts to the Organizational Structure

4.18 The chart of accounts must conform to the hospital organizational structure. Consider, for example, the partial organization chart in Figure 4-4. Assume that the activities of the hospital are organized into five major divisions:

- Nursing Services
- Other Professional (Ancillary) Services
- General (Support) Services
- Fiscal Services
- Administrative Services

Each division is composed of numerous organizational units (departments). The manager of each unit has a defined authority and responsibility to accomplish the mission of the unit. In doing so, the manager will make decisions and take actions that result in the incurring of expenses and, in some units, the generation of revenues. Each organizational unit is referred to as a *responsibility center*. All centers incur expenses, but some centers also generate revenues.

4.19 A close relationship must exist between the chart of accounts and the hospital's organizational structure. The chart of accounts must be designed so that each responsibility center has a series of accounts to record the expenses it incurs and (if it is a revenue-producing center) a series of accounts to record the revenues it earns. Budgeted revenues and expenses are also classified by these same responsibility centers. In this way, useful information is developed that facilitates managerial evaluation of the performance of each center and its manager.

4.20 In Figure 4-4, the correspondence between the chart of accounts and the organizational structure is illustrated. The hospital pharmacy, organized under the Other Professional Services Division, is an expense center and a revenue center. Its revenues are recorded in the 4-3700-00 series of accounts; its expenses are recorded in the 6-3700-00 series of accounts. The responsibility center code for the pharmacy is 3700.

4.21 The Housekeeping Department, organized under the General Services Division, is an expense center, but not a revenue center. The chart of accounts provides no revenue accounts for this department; its expenses are recorded in the 7-6300-00 series of accounts. The responsibility center code for housekeeping is 6300.

4.22 Figure 4-5 presents an illustrative outline of the primary income statement accounts, assuming a particular organizational structure. The indicated account numbers do not include either the primary prefix (the entity designator) or the secondary prefix (the fund designator). Further discussion of these accounts appears in Chapter 6.

Figure 4-4
Hospital Organization Chart (Partial)

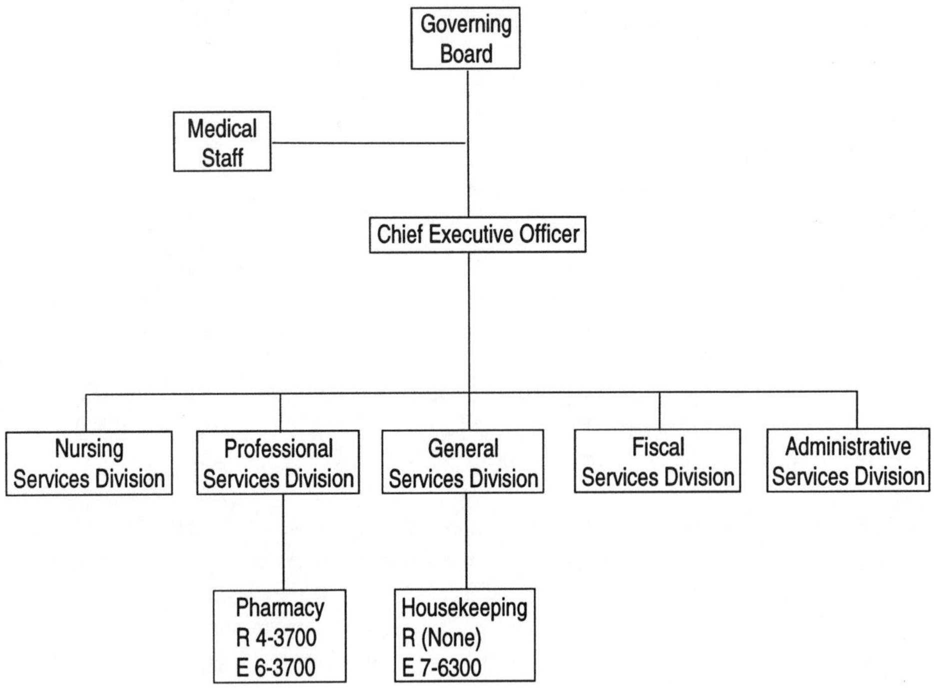

Figure 4-5

Outline of the Statement of Income and Other Changes in Unrestricted Equity Accounts

Account Numbers		
Expenses	Revenues	Account Titles
		NURSING SERVICES DIVISION
6-0100-00		Nursing Services, General
6-0110-00		Nursing—Administration
6-0115-00		Nursing—Staff Development and Education
6-0120-00		Float Nursing Personnel
6-0125-00		Central Transportation
6-0200-00	4-0200-00	Nursing Units—Medical and Surgical Acute
6–0210–00 to 6–0490–00	4–0210–00 to 4–0490–00	Designated Medical and Surgical Acute Care Units
6-0500-00	4-0500-00	Pediatric Acute
6-0600-00	4-0600-00	Psychiatric Acute
6-0700-00	4-0700-00	Obstetric (Gynecologic) Acute
6-0800-00	4-0800-00	Newborn Nursery Acute
6-0810-00	4-0810-00	Premature Units
6-0820-00	4-0820-00	Normal Delivery Units
6-0900-00	4-0900-00	Other Adult and Pediatric Acute Care Units
6-0910-00	4-0910-00	Detoxification Unit
6-0920-00	4-0920-00	Communicable Disease Unit
6-1200-00	4-1200-00	Intensive Care
6-1210-00	4-1210-00	Medical and Surgical Unit
6-1220-00	4-1220-00	Pediatric Unit
6-1230-00	4-1230-00	Neonatal Unit
6-1240-00	4-1240-00	Definitive Observation Unit
6-1250-00	4-1250-00	Psychiatric
6-1300-00	4-1300-00	Burn Care
6-1400-00	4-1400-00	Cardiac Care
6-1410-00	4-1410-00	Myocardial Infarction Unit
6-1420-00	4-1420-00	Pulmonary Unit
6-1430-00	4-1430-00	Heart Transplant Unit

Account Numbers		
Expenses	**Revenues**	**Account Titles**
6-1500-00	4-1500-00	Extended (Long-Term) and Other Nonacute Care Units
6-1510-00	4-1510-00	Skilled Nursing Unit
6-1520-00	4-1520-00	Rehabilitation Unit
6-1530-00	4-1530-00	Long-Term Psychiatric Unit
6-1540-00	4-1540-00	Residential Unit
6-1550-00	4-1550-00	Self-Care Unit
6-1600-00	4-1600-00	Hemodialysis
6-1700-00	4-1700-00	Respiratory Services
6-1710-00	4-1710-00	Respiratory Therapy
6-1720-00	4-1720-00	Pulmonary Function Testing
6-1900-00	4-1900-00	Labor and Delivery Services
6-1910-00	4-1910-00	Labor Rooms
6-1920-00	4-1920-00	Delivery Rooms
6-2100-00	4-2100-00	Surgical Services
6-2101-00		Administrative Office
6-2110-00	4-2110-00	General Surgery
6-2120-00	4-2120-00	Organ Transplants
6-2130-00	4-2130-00	Open-Heart Surgery
6-2140-00	4-2140-00	Neurosurgery
6-2150-00	4-2150-00	Orthopedic Surgery
6-2160-00	4-2160-00	Minor Surgery
6-2170-00	4-2170-00	Surgical Day Care (Mini-Surgery)
6-2180-00	4-2180-00	Recovery Rooms
6-2300-00	4-2300-00	Emergency and Ambulance Services
6-2301-00		Administrative Office
6-2310-00	4-2310-00	Emergency Department
6-2315-00	4-2315-00	Ambulance Service
6-2320-00	4-2320-00	Private Referred Ambulatory
6-2500-00	4-2500-00	Central Services and Supply
6-2510-00	4-2510-00	Central Services
6-2520-00	4-2520-00	Central Sterile Supply

Account Numbers		
Expenses	**Revenues**	**Account Titles**
		OTHER PROFESSIONAL SERVICES DIVISION
6-3100-00	4-3100-00	Laboratory Services
6-3110-00		Administrative Office
6-3115-00		Animal Maintenance
6-3120-00	4-3120-00	Autopsy
6-3125-00	4-3125-00	Blood Bank
6-3130-00	4-3130-00	Chemistry
6-3135-00	4-3135-00	Hematology
6-3140-00	4-3140-00	Histology
6-3145-00	4-3145-00	Immunology
6-3150-00	4-3150-00	Microbiology
6-3155-00		Procurement and Dispatch
6-3160-00	4-3160-00	Radioisotopes
6-3165-00	4-3165-00	Special Procedures
6-3270-00	4-3270-00	Urine and Feces
6-3300-00	4-3300-00	Electrodiagnosis
6-3310-00		Administrative Office
6-3320-00	4-3320-00	Electrocardiology
6-3330-00	4-3330-00	Electromyography
6-3340-00	4-3340-00	Electrocephalography
6-3400-00	4-3400-00	Radiology—Diagnostic
6-3410-00		Administrative Office
6-3420-00	4-3420-00	Angiocardiography
6-3500-00	4-3500-00	Radiology—Therapeutic
6-3510-00		Administrative Office
6-3520-00	4-3520-00	Chemotherapy
6-3530-00	4-3530-00	Radiation Therapy
6-3600-00	4-3600-00	Nuclear Medicine
6-3610-00		Administrative Office
6-3620-00	4-3620-00	Diagnostic
6-3630-00	4-3630-00	Therapeutic
6-3700-00	4-3700-00	Pharmacy
6-3800-00	4-3800-00	Anesthesiology
6-3900-00	4-3900-00	Rehabilitation Services

Account Numbers		
Expenses	**Revenues**	**Account Titles**
6-3910-00		Administrative Office
6-3920-00	4-3920-00	Physical Therapy
6-3930-00	4-3930-00	Occupational Therapy
6-3940-00	4-3940-00	Speech Therapy
6-3950-00	4-3950-00	Recreational Therapy
6-4100-00	4-4100-00	Clinic Services
6-4110-00		Administrative Office
6-4115-00	4-4115-00	Cardiology Clinic
6-4120-00	4-4120-00	Eye, Ear, Nose, and Throat Clinic
6-4125-00	4-4125-00	Medical and Surgical Clinic
6-4130-00	4-4130-00	Obstetrics and Gynecology Clinic
6-4135-00	4-4135-00	Orthopedics Clinic
6-4140-00	4-4140-00	Pediatrics Clinic
6-4145-00	4-4145-00	Physical Medicine Clinic
6-4150-00	4-4150-00	Psychiatric Clinic
6-4155-00	4-4155-00	Urology Clinic
6-4300-00	4-4300-00	Home Care
6-4310-00		Administrative Office
6-4320-00	4-4320-00	Hospice
6-4330-00	4-4330-00	Nursing Service
6-4340-00	4-4340-00	Rehabilitation Service
6-4400-00	4-4400-00	Social Services
6-4500-00		Health Records and Library Services
6-4510-00		Health Records
6-4520-00		Medical Library
		DEDUCTIONS FROM REVENUES
		(Note: These accounts are used only for purposes of internal accounting. See paragraph 4.8.)
5-1100-00		Contractual Adjustments
5-1110-00		Medicare Standard Arrangement
5-1120-00		Public Aid Programs
5-1130-00		Charge-Based Third Parties
5-1140-00		Third-Party Risk Arrangements

Account Numbers		
Expenses	**Revenues**	**Account Titles**
5-1200-00		Charity Services
5-1300-00		Other Revenue Deductions
5-1310-00		Courtesy Discounts
5-1320-00		Administrative Adjustments
		OTHER REVENUES AND ASSETS RELEASED FROM RESTRICTIONS
	5-2100-00	Tuition
	5-2110-00	School of Nursing
	5-2120-00	Licensed Vocational Nurse Program
	5-2130-00	Paramedical Education
	5-2140-00	Interns
	5-2150-00	Residents
	5-3000-00	Cafeteria
	5-3100-00	Laundry and Linen Services
	5-3200-00	Communication Services
	5-3300-00	Parking
	5-3400-00	Television and Radio Rentals
	5-3500-00	Health (Medical) Record and Abstract Fees
	5-3600-00	Sales of Scrap and Waste
	5-3700-00	Vending Machine Commissions
	5-4000-00	Rentals
	5-4010-00	Student Housing
	5-4020-00	Employee Housing
	5-4030-00	Nonpatient Rooms
	5-4040-00	Physicians' Offices
	5-4100-00	Donated Services and Commodities
	5-4110-00	Donated Services
	5-4120-00	Donated Commodities
	5-4200-00	Cash Discounts, Rebates, and Refunds from Vendors
	5-5000-00	Services to Other Entities
	5-5010-00	Purchasing
	5-5020-00	Janitorial
	5-5030-00	Laundry and Linen

Account Numbers		
Expenses	**Revenues**	**Account Titles**
	5-5040-00	Education
	5-5050-00	Management
	5-5060-00	Data Processing
	5-5070-00	Research Fees and Royalties
	5-6000-00	Grants and Tax Appropriations
	5-6100-00	Grants
	5-6200-00	Tax Appropriations
	5-9000-00	Assets Released from Donor Restrictions
	5-9100-00	Satisfaction of Specific-Purpose Restrictions
	5-9200-00	Satisfaction of Equipment Acquisition Restrictions
	5-9300-00	Satisfaction of Time Restrictions
		GENERAL SERVICES DIVISION
7-6000-00		Dietary
7-6010-00		Administrative Office
7-6020-00		Kitchen
7-6030-00		Patient Food Service
7-6040-00		Cafeteria
7-6100-00		Plant Operation
7-6110-00		Administrative Office
7-6120-00		Grounds
7-6130-00		Boiler and Power Plant
7-6140-00		Parking
7-6150-00		Elevator Operation
7-6160-00		Security
7-6200-00		Plant Maintenance
7-6210-00		Administrative Office
7-6220-00		Carpentry
7-6230-00		Plumbing
7-6240-00		Painting
7-6250-00		Electrical and Refrigeration
7-6260-00		Automotive
7-6300-00		Housekeeping

Account Numbers		
Expenses	**Revenues**	**Account Titles**
7-6400-00		Laundry and Linen Service
7-6410-00		Laundry
7-6420-00		Linen
		FISCAL AND ADMINISTRATIVE SERVICES DIVISION
7-7000-00		Fiscal Services
7-7010-00		Administrative Office
7-7015-00		General Accounting
7-7020-00		Budgets and Costs
7-7025-00		Payroll Accounting
7-7030-00		Accounts Payable Accounting
7-7035-00		Plant and Equipment Accounting
7-7040-00		Inventory Accounting
7-7045-00		Patients' Accounts
7-7050-00		Admitting
7-7055-00		Cashiering
7-7060-00		Credit and Collections
7-8000-00		Administrative Services
7-8010-00		Administrative Office
7-8015-00		Governing Board
7-8020-00		Auxiliary Groups
7-8025-00		Chaplaincy Services
7-8030-00		Public Relations and Development
7-8035-00		Purchasing
7-8040-00		Communications
7-8045-00		Information Services
7-8050-00		Printing and Duplicating
7-8055-00		Receiving and Stores
7-8060-00		Personnel
7-8065-00		Employee Medical Services
7-8070-00		Medical Care Evaluation

Account Numbers		
Expenses	**Revenues**	**Account Titles**
		RESEARCH AND EDUCATION
8-1000-00		Research
8-1010-00		Administrative Office
8-1200-00		Hospital Research Projects
8-1300-00		Joint Research Projects
8-1400-00		Medical School Research Projects
8-4000-00		Education
8-4010-00		Administrative Office
8-4100-00		Nursing and Allied Health Education
8-4110-00		Administrative Office
8-4115-00		Registered Nurse Program
8-4120-00		Licensed Practical Nurse Program
8-4125-00		Allied Health Education
8-4200-00		Graduate Medical Education
8-4210-00		Voluntary Medical Staff
8-4215-00		Paid Medical Staff
8-4220-00		Interns
8-4225-00		Residents
		UNASSIGNED EXPENSES
		(Unassigned expenses, sometimes called indirect expenses, are those whose direct assignment to responsibility centers in the regular accounting process is impractical or inconvenient.)
8-6100-00		Depreciation
8-6182-00		Land Improvements
8-6183-00		Buildings
8-6184-00		Leasehold Improvements
8-6185-00		Fixed Equipment
8-6186-00		Major Movable Equipment
8-6200-00		Rent
8-6300-00		Insurance

Account Numbers		
Expenses	**Revenues**	**Account Titles**
8-6400-00		Interest
8-6410-00		Working Capital Interest
8-6415-00		Other Interest
8-7100-00		Employee Benefits
8-7110-00		Social Security Taxes
8-7115-00		Federal and State Unemployment Taxes
8-7120-00		Group Health and Life Insurance
8-7125-00		Retirement Plan Expense
8-7130-00		Workmen's Compensation Insurance
8-7135-00		Group Disability Insurance
8-7200-00		Housing
8-7210-00		Students
8-7215-00		Employees
8-7220-00		Physicians' Offices
8-7300-00		Medical Photography and Illustration
8-7400-00		Medical Malpractice Expense
8-8000-00		Taxes
8-8100-00		Income Tax Expense
8-8110-00		Federal Income Tax Expense Currently Payable
8-8115-00		Provision for Deferred Federal Income Tax
8-8120-00		State Income Tax Expense Currently Payable
8-8125-00		Provision for Deferred State Income Tax
8-8200-00		Property Tax Expense
8-8300-00		Payments in Lieu of Taxes
		NONOPERATING GAINS AND LOSSES (Depending on the hospital's definition of its ongoing major or central activities, certain of the following accounts may be appropriately classified as other revenues or operating gains.)
	9-1000-00	Unrestricted Contributions
	9-2000-00	Income and Gains (Losses) on Investments
	9-2100-00	Investments of Unrestricted Resources
	9-2200-00	Investments of Restricted Resources

Account Numbers		
Expenses	**Revenues**	**Account Titles**
	9-2300-00	Investments Whose Use Is Limited
	9-3000-00	Gains (Losses) on Disposal of Plant Assets
		OTHER ACCOUNTS
	9-9100-00	Gain (Loss) on Disposal of a Business Segment
	9-9200-00	Extraordinary Gains (Losses)
	9-9300-00	Cumulative Effect on Prior Years of Change in Accounting Principle

5

Balance Sheet and Statement of Changes in Equity Accounts

5.1 A balance sheet is a financial statement that reflects, at a given date, the financial position of an enterprise in terms of its assets, liabilities, and equity (fund balances, where fund accounting is used). (Definitions of the terms *assets, liabilities,* and *equity* appear in Chapter 2.) A statement of changes in equity (both unrestricted and restricted) summarizes the increases and decreases in equity during a specified period of time. The specific accounts needed for the accumulation of information for these financial statement presentations are described in this chapter. The account numbers indicated generally do not include either the primary prefix (entity designator) or the secondary prefix (fund designator).

CURRENT ASSETS

5.2 Current assets consist of cash and other assets commonly identified as those that are reasonably expected to be converted into cash or sold or consumed within one year or within the operating cycle, whichever is longer. (The hospital operating cycle generally is less than one year.)[1] If cash, investments, and other assets are being held for the acquisition of plant assets or for liquidation of long-term debt, however, those assets usually are classified as noncurrent.

1 Accounting Research Bulletin No. 43: *Restatement and Revision of Accounting Research Bulletins* (New York: Accounting Principles Board, 1953), Chapter 3, Section A, Paragraph 4.

5.3 Cash and Cash Equivalents

1-1000-00	Cash
1-1100-00	General Checking Accounts
1-1110-00	Bank #1
1-1120-00	Bank #2
1-1200-00	Payroll Checking Accounts
1-1300-00	Other Checking Accounts
1-1400-00	Imprest Cash Funds
1-1410-00	Petty Cash Funds
1-1420-00	Check Cashing Funds
1-1500-00	Savings Accounts
1-1600-00	Certificates of Deposit
1-1700-00	U.S. Treasury Bills and Notes
1-1900-00	Assets Whose Use Is Limited and Required for Payment of Current Liabilities (see paragraph 5.12)

These accounts for cash and cash equivalents represent the amount of cash on deposit in banks that is immediately available for use, the amount of cash on hand for minor disbursements, and the amount of cash invested in savings accounts, certificates of deposit, U.S. Treasury bills and notes, or similar cash equivalents.

5.4 Short-Term Investments

1-2000-00	Short-Term Investments
1-2100-00	Government Securities
1-2110-00	U.S. Treasury Bonds
1-2120-00	State and Municipal Bonds
1-2200-00	Corporate Bonds
1-2300-00	Corporate Stocks
1-2310-00	Common Stocks
1-2320-00	Preferred Stocks

Purchases of short-term investments in governmental and corporate securities, evidenced by certificates of ownership or indebtedness, are recorded at acquisition cost. Donated securities should be recorded at their fair market value at the date of donation. At each reporting date, marketable equity securities generally should be adjusted to their current market values in accordance with FAS 115.[2] If there is an intent and an ability to hold marketable debt securities to maturity, however, those securities should be carried at amortized cost.

5.5 Receivables—Patients

1-3000-00	Receivables—Patient-Specific
1-3100-00	Inpatient Receivables
1-3110-00	Inhouse
1-3120-00	Discharged—Unbilled
1-3130-00	Discharged—Billed—Medicare Standard Arrangement
1-3140-00	Discharged—Billed—Public Aid Programs
1-3150-00	Discharged—Billed—Charge-Based Third Parties
1-3160-00	Discharged—Billed—Third-Party Risk Arrangements
1-3170-00	Discharged—Billed—Other Third Parties
1-3180-00	Discharged—Billed—Self-Pay
1-3200-00	Outpatient Receivables
1-3220-00	Unbilled
1-3230-00	Billed—Medicare Standard Arrangement
1-3240-00	Billed—Public Aid Programs
1-3250-00	Billed—Charge-Based Third Parties
1-3260-00	Billed—Third-Party Risk Arrangements
1-3270-00	Billed—Other Third Parties
1-3280-00	Billed—Self-Pay

The accounts in the 1-3000-00 to 1-3290-00 series should reflect all unpaid amounts for hospital services provided to inpatients and outpatients. These accounts are identified by primary payer as set forth in Principles and Practices Board Statement No. 16, *Classifying, Valuing, and Analyzing Accounts Receivable Related to Patient Services,* as follows:

1. Medicare standard arrangement;
2. Public aid programs, including Medicaid (Title XIX of the Social Security Act), Aid to Dependent Children, and similar state and local programs;
3. Charge-based payments by third parties, such as commercial insurance;

2 Statement of Financial Accounting Standards No. 115, *Accounting for Certain Investments in Debt and Equity Securities* (Norwalk, Connecticut: FASB, 1993).

4. Risk arrangements with third parties, such as health maintenance organizations (HMO), comprehensive medical plans (CMP), and similar arrangements in which the provider shares risk with the insurer and in which an individual patient-specific payment amount can be identified. Third-party risk arrangements may be sponsored by Medicare, Medicaid, Blue Cross, commercial insurance companies, unions, and others;

5. Third parties other than those specified above, such as preferred provider organizations (PPO), worker compensation programs, Indian Health Service, and CHAMPUS; and

6. Self-pay, which includes only those services for which a patient has no third-party payment arrangement or plans to handle the relations with a third-party payer personally, and therefore is personally liable for the services rendered.

If desired, the two-digit suffix may be used to obtain a more detailed classification such as identifying specific public aid programs. The nature of this further classification is determined by the informational requirements of the individual hospital.

5.6 Allowance for Uncollectible Receivables

1-3300-00	Allowance for Uncollectible Receivables
1-3310-00	Bad Debts
1-3320-00	Contractual Adjustments
1-3330-00	Charity Service
1-3340-00	Courtesy Discounts
1-3350-00	Other

The accounts in the 1-3300-00 series are valuation (or contra-asset) accounts whose credit balances represent the estimated amount of uncollectible receivables from patients and their third-party sponsors. A more detailed classification can be maintained by the use of the two-digit suffix. For example, the first digit of the two-digit suffix can be used to denote type of patient, i.e., "1" for inpatient and "2" for outpatient. The second digit may be used for another purpose.

5.7 Other Receivables

1-4000-00	Other Receivables
1-4100-00	Due from Third-Party Payers
1-4200-00	Pledges Receivable
1-4250-00	Allowance for Uncollectible Pledges
1-4300-00	Grants and Legacies Receivable

1-4400-00	Due from Staff and Employees
1-4500-00	Due from Affiliated Organizations
1-4600-00	Due from Other Funds
1-4700-00	Accrued Interest Receivable
1-4800-00	Dividends Receivable
1-4900-00	Other

The accounts in the 1-4100-00 series reflect the amounts due from third-party reimbursement programs based on cost reports submitted and/or audited. Subaccounts can be maintained for each year's settlement where more than one year's settlement is uncollected. The accounts in the 1-4200-00 to 1-4900-00 series reflect the amounts due from various sources for other than patient services.

5.8 Other Current Assets

1-5000-00	Other Current Assets
1-5100-00	Inventory
1-5110-00	General Stores
1-5120-00	Pharmacy
1-5130-00	Central Supply
1-5140-00	Dietary
1-5150-00	Plant Operation and Maintenance
1-5190-00	Other
1-5200-00	Prepaid Expenses
1-5210-00	Insurance
1-5220-00	Interest
1-5230-00	Rent
1-5240-00	Pension Plan Expense
1-5290-00	Other
1-5300-00	Deferred Income Taxes
1-5400-00	Deferred Third-Party Debits

The inventory accounts reflect the cost of unused hospital supplies. Inventories may be valued by any generally accepted method (FIFO, LIFO, average cost), but the method used must be applied consistently from year to year. Where feasible, perpetual inventory records should be maintained and adjusted periodically to physical count. The extent of inventory control and detailed record keeping will depend on unit costs, quantities purchased and used, susceptibility to theft, and other factors.

5.9 The prepaid expense accounts reflect incurred costs that are properly chargeable to a future accounting period. If material, amounts that are prepaid for more than one year should be reported as noncurrent assets.

NONCURRENT ASSETS

5.10 Noncurrent assets include long-term investments, assets whose use is limited or restricted, plant and equipment, and certain other assets.

5.11 Long-Term Investments

1-6000-00	Long-Term Investments
1-6100-00	Government Securities
1-6110-00	U.S. Government Bonds
1-6120-00	State and Municipal Bonds
1-6200-00	Corporate Bonds
1-6300-00	Corporate Stocks
1-6310-00	Preferred Stocks
1-6320-00	Common Stocks
1-6400-00	Investments in Affiliated Entities

Purchased investments in debt and equity securities initially are recorded at acquisition cost. Securities acquired by donation should be recorded at fair market value at date of receipt. Except for investments that are accounted for by the equity method, long-term investments in equity and debt securities generally should be adjusted to fair market value at each reporting date. However, long-term investments in debt securities are carried at amortized cost if there is an intent and an ability to hold those securities until maturity.

5.12 Assets Whose Use Is Limited or Restricted

1-7000-00	Assets Whose Use Is Limited or Restricted
1-7100-00	By Board for Capital Improvements
1-7200-00	By Third-Party Payers for Funded Depreciation
1-7300-00	By Malpractice Funding Arrangement—Held by Trustee
1-7400-00	By Bond Indenture—Held by Trustee
1-7500-00	By Donors for Specific Operating Purposes
1-7600-00	By Donors for Plant Replacement and Expansion Purposes

1-7700-00	By Donors for Term Endowment Purposes
1-7800-00	By Donors for Permanent Endowment Purposes
1-7900-00	Assets Whose Use Is Limited— Reclassified to Current Assets

The accounts in the 1-7000-00 series represent the amounts of assets whose use is *limited* (by action of the hospital's board of directors or by contract with third-party payers, bondholders, or other external parties) or *restricted* by donors. Appropriate subaccounts should be maintained according to the needs of the individual hospital. These assets generally are in the form of cash, interest and dividends receivable, and investments. Amounts that are required for the payment of current liabilities should be reclassified and reported as current assets as illustrated in Figure 7-1.

5.13 Property, Plant, and Equipment

1-8000-00	Property, Plant, and Equipment
1-8100-00	Land
1-8200-00	Land Improvements
1-8300-00	Buildings
1-8400-00	Leasehold Improvements
1-8500-00	Fixed Equipment
1-8600-00	Major Movable Equipment
1-8700-00	Minor Equipment
1-8800-00	Construction in Progress
1-8900-00	Accumulated Depreciation
1-8982-00	Land Improvements
1-8983-00	Buildings
1-8984-00	Leasehold Improvements
1-8985-00	Fixed Equipment
1-8986-00	Major Movable Equipment

The accounts in the 1-8100-00 series reflect the cost of land used in hospital operations. Included here are the costs of off-site sewer and water lines, charges for installing public utilities, street paving, and sewers, and permanent roadways and grading of a nondepreciable nature, curbs and sidewalks whose replacement is not the responsibility of the hospital, and other land expenditures of a nondepreciable nature. Unlike buildings and equipment, land does not deteriorate with use nor with the passage of time; therefore, land is nondepreciable.

5.14 The accounts in the 1-8200-00 series are used to record the cost of depreciable land improvements. This includes the costs of on-site sewer and water lines; paving of roadways, parking lots, curbs, and sidewalks (if replacement is the responsibility of the hospital); and the cost of shrubbery, fences, and walls.

5.15 The accounts in the 1-8300-00 series reflect the cost of all buildings (and the cost of any subsequent additions and improvements) used in hospital operations. This includes architectural, consulting, and legal fees related to the acquisition or construction of buildings. Interest costs incurred during the construction period may also be capitalized as a part of the cost of buildings.[3]

5.16 The accounts in the 1-8400-00 series are charged with the cost of all depreciable improvements of leased land and buildings used in hospital operations. Detailed property and depreciation records usually are maintained for these accounts.

5.17 All expenditures for fixed equipment are recorded in the accounts in the 1-8500-00 series. Fixed equipment has the following general characteristics:

- Affixed to the building and not subject to removal and transfer;
- A life of more than three years, but less than that of the building to which it is affixed; and
- Used in hospital operations.

Fixed equipment includes such items as boilers, generators, elevators, incinerators, engines, pumps, air conditioning systems, and refrigeration machinery. Detailed subsidiary property and depreciation records usually are maintained for these accounts.

5.18 The accounts in the 1-8600-00 series are used to record the cost of major movable equipment used in hospital operations. Major movable equipment has the following general characteristics:

- Movable, as distinguished from fixed equipment;
- Occupies a more or less fixed location in the building;
- Unit cost large enough to justify the expense incident to control by means of an equipment subsidiary ledger;
- Sufficient individuality and size to make control feasible by means of identification tags;
- Minimum life of three years or more; and
- Used in hospital operations.

3 Statement of Financial Accounting Standards No. 34, *Capitalization of Interest Cost* (Norwalk, Connecticut: FASB, 1979).

Examples of major movable equipment are such items as automobiles and trucks, desks, beds, chairs, computers, operating tables, oxygen tents, sterilizers, and X-ray apparatus. Detailed subsidiary property and depreciation records usually are maintained for these accounts.

5.19 The accounts in the 1-8700-00 series are used to record the cost of minor equipment used in hospital operations. Minor equipment has the following general characteristics:

- Location generally not fixed, it is subject to requisition or use by various departments of the hospital;
- Relatively small size;
- Subject to storeroom control;
- Fairly large number in use;
- Useful life generally three years or less; and
- Used in hospital operations.

Minor equipment includes such items as wastebaskets, bed pans, basins, glassware, silverware, pots and pans, mattresses, and surgical instruments.

5.20 Accounts in the 1-8800-00 series should be used to accumulate the costs of construction during the construction period. Upon completion of the construction program, these accounts should be closed out and the accumulated costs should be transferred to the appropriate plant asset accounts.

5.21 Accounts in the 1-8900-00 series reflect the amount of depreciation accumulated on the hospital's depreciable assets. As indicated, separate accumulated depreciation accounts are maintained for each major category of depreciable assets. Any generally accepted depreciation method (such as the straight-line, productivity, sum-of-years'-digits, and declining-balance methods) may be used for each asset or group of assets, but the selected methods adopted should be used consistently from year to year.

5.22 Other Noncurrent Assets

1-9000-00	Other Noncurrent Assets
1-9100-00	Nonoperating Plant Assets
1-9200-00	Accumulated Depreciation—Nonoperating Plant Assets
1-9300-00	Deferred Financing Costs
1-9400-00	Intangible Assets
1-9410-00	Goodwill

1-9420-00	Other
1-9500-00	Deferred Income Taxes
1-9600-00	Deferred Third-Party Debits

Accounts in the 1-9100-00 series are used to record the cost of investments in plant assets not used in hospital operations, including medical office buildings. Accumulated depreciation on these plant assets is recorded in the 1-9200-00 series of accounts.

5.23 Deferred financing costs, such as bond issue costs, are charged to the accounts in the 1-9300-00 series. Bond issue costs are amortized to expense over the term of the bonds. The cost of intangible assets, such as goodwill, are charged to the accounts in the 1-9400-00 series. Intangible assets should be amortized to expense in accordance with APB Opinion No. 17.[4]

CURRENT LIABILITIES

5.24 Current liabilities are obligations whose liquidation is reasonably expected to require the use of resources properly classified as current assets, or the creation of other current liabilities. A primary concept is that current liabilities are those that mature within one year or the operating cycle, whichever is longer.[5]

5.25 Current Maturities of Long-term Debt

2-1000-00	Current Maturities of Long-Term Debt
2-1081-00	Mortgages Payable
2-1082-00	Notes Payable
2-1083-00	Bonds Payable
2-1084-00	Obligation under Capital Leases

Accounts in the 2-1000-00 series are used to record the portion of mortgages, notes, bonds, and other long-term debt that matures within one year and is reportable as a current liability.

5.26 Short-Term Notes and Loans Payable

2-2000-00	Short-Term Notes and Loans Payable
2-2100-00	Banks

4 APB Opinion No. 17, *Intangible Assets* (New York: AICPA, 1970).

5 Statement of Financial Accounting Standards No. 6, *Classification of Short-Term Obligations Expected to Be Refinanced* (Norwalk, Connecticut: FASB, 1975), paragraph 2.

2-2200-00	Vendors
2-2300-00	Others

Accounts in the 2-2000-00 series are used to record obligations in the form of promissory notes owed to banks, vendors, and others.

5.27 Accounts Payable

2-3000-00	Accounts Payable
2-3100-00	Trade Accounts
2-3200-00	Other Accounts

Accounts in the 2-3000-0 series are used to record the amounts owed to suppliers and other creditors for supplies, equipment, and services purchased on open account.

5.28 Accrued Employee Compensation and Related Liabilities

2-4000-00	Accrued Employee Compensation and Related Liabilities
2-4100-00	Accrued Payroll
2-4200-00	Accrued Vacation, Holiday, and Sick Pay
2-4300-00	Taxes Withheld and Accrued
2-4310-00	Income Taxes
2-4320-00	Social Security Taxes
2-4400-00	Unemployment Taxes Payable
2-4500-00	Accrued Workmen's Compensation Insurance
2-4600-00	Accrued Hospitalization Insurance Premiums
2-4700-00	Union Dues Payable
2-4800-00	Accrued Pension Plan Liability
2-4900-00	Obligation for Other Postemployment Benefits

Accounts in the 2-4000-00 series are used to record the actual or estimated liabilities of the hospital for salaries and wages earned by employees, and for taxes and other payroll-related obligations.

5.29 Other Accrued Expenses Payable

2-5000-00	Other Accrued Expenses Payable
2-5100-00	Interest
2-5200-00	Rent
2-5300-00	Property Taxes
2-5400-00	Fees Payable to Medical Specialists
2-5500-00	Current Portion of Estimated Malpractice Costs

Accounts in the 2-5000-00 series are used to record various other expenses that have been incurred but remain unpaid at the end of the reporting period.

5.30 Deferred Credits

2-6000-00	Deferred Credits
2-6100-00	Deferred Income
2-6200-00	Deferred Income Taxes
2-6300-00	Deferred Third-Party Revenue
2-6400-00	Patients' Deposits
2-6500-00	Unidentified Receipts
2-6600-00	Patients' Credit Balances

Accounts in the 2-6000-00 series are used to record a variety of deferred credits such as income received in advance, deferred income taxes and third-party revenues arising from timing differences that will reverse within one year, and unidentified receipts. Standards of accounting and reporting for deferred third-party revenue are set forth in the HFMA's Principles and Practices Board Statement No. 13, *Timing Differences Pertaining to Third-Party Payment.*

5.31 Other Current Liabilities

2-7000-00	Other Current Liabilities
2-7100-00	Advances from Third-Party Payers
2-7200-00	Due to Third-Party Payers
2-7300-00	Dividends Payable
2-7400-00	Income Taxes Payable
2-7500-00	Due to Affiliated Entities
2-7600-00	Due to Other Funds
2-7700-00	Construction Contracts Payable

Accounts in the 2-7000-00 series are used to record those current liabilities for which accounts have not been provided elsewhere.

NONCURRENT LIABILITIES

5.32 Noncurrent liabilities consist of various forms of long-term debt, deferred credits, and certain other obligations.

5.33 Long-Term Debt

2-8000-00	Long-Term Debt
2-8100-00	Mortgages Payable
2-8200-00	Notes Payable
2-8300-00	Bonds Payable
2-8310-00	Term Bonds Payable
2-8320-00	Serial Bonds Payable
2-8380-00	Unamortized Bond Premium
2-8390-00	Unamortized Bond Discount
2-8400-00	Obligation under Capital Leases
2-8500-00	Pension Plan Liability
2-8600-00	Other Postretirement Benefits Liability

Accounts in the 2-8000-00 series are used to record noncurrent liabilities evidenced by formal contracts such as mortgages, promissory notes, bond indentures, leases, and pension plans. Pertinent financial accounting standards appear in pronouncements such as APB Opinion No. 21, *Interest on Receivables and Payables,* FAS No. 13, *Accounting for Leases,* FAS No. 87, *Employers' Accounting for Pension Plans,* and FAS No. 106, *Employers' Accounting for Postretirement Benefits other than Pensions.*

5.34 Other Noncurrent Liabilities

2-9000-00	Other Noncurrent Liabilities
2-9100-00	Deferred Credits
2-9110-00	Deferred Income
2-9120-00	Deferred Income Taxes
2-9130-00	Deferred Third-Party Revenue
2-9200-00	Estimated Malpractice Costs

Accounts in the 2-9000-00 series are used to record the hospital's noncurrent liabilities other than those properly includible in the 2-8000-00 series of accounts.

EQUITY

5.35 The equity, or net assets, of investor-owned and not-for-profit hospitals is the difference between total assets and total liabilities. Equity is increased by revenues and gains, and is decreased by expenses and losses. An investor-owned hospital's equity also may be increased by investments of assets by owners, and it may be decreased by distributions of assets to its owners. Similarly, the equity of a not-for-profit hospital may be increased by the receipt of assets from donors who may impose temporary or permanent restrictions on their use.

5.36 The equity accounts of an investor-owned hospital are substantially the same as those employed by other investor-owned entities. The equity accounts of a not-for-profit hospital are considerably different.

Equity of Not-for-Profit Hospitals

5.37 This illustrative chart of accounts provides the following equity accounts for the not-for-profit hospital:

3-1000-00	**Equity—Unrestricted**
3-1100-00	Income Summary
3-1200-00	Interequity Reclassifications
3-1300-00	Prior Period Adjustments
	Equity—Temporarily Donor-Restricted
3-2000-00	For Specific Operating Purposes
3-2100-00	Contributions Received
3-2200-00	Investment Income, Gains, and Losses
3-2300-00	Interequity Reclassifications
3-3000-00	For Plant Replacement and Expansion
3-3100-00	Contributions Received
3-3200-00	Investment Income, Gains, and Losses
3-3300-00	Interequity Reclassifications
3-4000-00	For Term Endowments
3-4100-00	Contributions Received
3-4200-00	Investment Income Gains, and Losses
3-4300-00	Interequity Reclassifications

3-5000-00	**Equity—Permanently Donor-Restricted**
3-5100-00	Contributions Received
3-5200-00	Investment Gains and Losses

5.38 The not-for-profit hospital's equity is divided into three major classes: (1) unrestricted equity, (2) temporarily restricted equity, and (3) permanently restricted equity. Temporarily restricted equity, in turn, is divided into three subclasses corresponding to the nature of the donor-imposed restrictions: specific operating purposes, acquisitions of plant assets, and term (time-restricted) endowments. A chart of accounts should provide for these classes of equity whether or not fund accounting and reporting is employed.

5.39 When fund accounting and reporting is followed by a not-for-profit hospital, however, the asset, liability, and equity account numbers will include the two-digit secondary prefix (see Chapter 4, paragraph 7) to designate the fund classification of each account. In addition, the titles of the primary equity accounts usually are modified as indicated below:

10-3-1000-00	Unrestricted (General) Fund Balance
20-3-2000-00	Specific Purposes Fund Balance
30-3-3000-00	Plant Replacement and Expansion Fund Balance
40-3-4000-00	Term Endowment Fund Balance
50-3-5000-00	Permanent Endowment Fund Balance

The term "fund balance," rather than "equity," generally is used in fund accounting and reporting. The Unrestricted Fund Balance is the hospital's unrestricted equity. The total of the Specific Purpose Fund Balance, the Plant Replacement and Expansion Fund Balance, and the Term Endowment Fund Balance is the hospital's temporarily restricted equity. The Permanent Endowment Fund Balance is the hospital's permanently donor-restricted fund balance.

5.40 The equity (fund balance) subaccounts are substantially the same whether or not fund accounting is employed. These subaccounts provide the information needed for preparation of statements of changes in equity:

3-1100-00 Income Summary

This account (in the annual closing of the books) is debited for the hospital's expenses and losses, and is credited for the hospital's revenues, gains, and other support, reflecting the change in unrestricted equity for the year. This account is used only in connection with unrestricted equity.

3–2100–00 3–3100–00 3–4100–00	Contributions Received

These accounts are credited for temporarily donor-restricted resources received by the hospital for specific operating purposes, for plant replacement and expansion, and for term endowments. These accounts are used only in connection with temporarily donor-restricted equity.

3-5100-00 Contributions Received

This account is credited for permanently donor-restricted resources received by the hospital for the establishment of permanent endowments. This account is used only in connection with permanently donor-restricted equity.

3–2200–00 3–3200–00	Investment Income, Gains, and Losses

These equity subaccounts are credited for investment income (interest and dividends), gains, and losses arising from investments of temporarily donor-restricted resources. If the investment income is not donor-restricted, however, the income is recorded as other revenues (or gains) and is reported in the hospital's statement of income and other changes in unrestricted equity.

No account for investment income is provided for temporarily or permanently donor-restricted equity related to term or permanent endowments because such income should be recorded as unrestricted revenues (or gains) or as increases in other temporarily donor-restricted equity (specific operating purpose or plant replacement and expansion), depending upon donor stipulations.

In current practice, gains (losses) arising from sales of investments of restricted resources generally are recorded as increases (decreases) in restricted equity, rather than as gains (losses) to be reported in the hospital's statement of income and other changes in unrestricted equity. (State laws differ on this matter.)

3-1300-00 Interequity Reclassifications

This account is debited for reclassifications of unrestricted equity to restricted equity. A donor, for example, may make a restricted contribution that requires a matching amount from the hospital. Reclassifications of restricted equity to unrestricted equity are not recorded in this account, but are recorded as credits to "assets released from restrictions" (account 5-9000-00).

3–2300–00 3–3300–00 3–4300–00	Interequity Reclassifications

These accounts are debited for reclassifications of restricted equity to unrestricted equity, and are credited for reclassifications of unrestricted equity to restricted equity.

For example, assume that donor restrictions on certain restricted resources are fulfilled. An entry is made to reclassify the resources from "Assets Whose Use Is Restricted" to the appropriate unrestricted asset category. A second entry is made, debiting the appropriate restricted interequity reclassifications account and crediting "Assets Released from Donor Restrictions."

3-1500-00 Prior Period Adjustments

This account is debited (credited) for prior period adjustments that arise from current period corrections of accounting errors made in prior periods that resulted in the misstatement of the income of those prior periods. In the current period, these adjustments are reported in the statement of income and other changes in unrestricted equity. Accounting and reporting guidance on this matter appears in APB Opinion No. 20, *Accounting Changes.*

Equity of Investor-Owned Hospital Corporations

3-6000-00	Stockholders' Equity
3-6100-00	Capital Stock
3-6200-00	Additional Contributed Capital
3-6300-00	Retained Earnings
3-6310-00	Prior Period Adjustments
3-6320-00	Income Summary
3-6330-00	Dividends Paid
3-6400-00	Treasury Stock

5.41 The equity of an investor-owned hospital corporation generally is referred to as *stockholders' equity*. Subaccounts in the 3-6000-00 series are used to record the amount invested in the corporation by its stockholders, the corporation's retained earnings, and changes in the retained earnings.

Equity of Investor-Owned Hospital Partnerships

3-7000-00	Partners' Equity
3-7100-00	Income Summary
3-7200-00	Partners' Drawings

5.42 The equity of an investor-owned hospital partnership generally is referred to as *partners' equity*. Subaccounts are used to record changes in the equity of each partner.

6

Statement of Income and Other Changes in Unrestricted Equity Accounts

6.1 The statement of income and other changes in unrestricted equity presents the increase (or decrease) in the hospital's unrestricted equity in terms of revenues earned, expenses incurred, gains, losses, and assets released from restrictions during a given period of time. As noted in Chapter 4, paragraph 19, revenues and *direct* expenses should be classified primarily according to the responsibility centers in which the revenues are generated and the expenses are incurred.[1] Revenues and expenses also should be subclassified (using the two-digit suffix) in some useful manner as illustrated in Figures 4-2 and 4-3. In addition, the chart of accounts should be designed to provide the classifications of revenues and expenses that may be needed for special-purpose reporting.

1 A "direct expense," such as the salary of an employee who works solely in one department, is one that is readily identifiable with a particular responsibility center and is subject to control by the center manager. An "indirect expense," such as depreciation of the hospital building, is one that is identifiable with many responsibility centers and is not subject to control by the manager of any center.

REVENUES AND EXPENSES—PATIENT SERVICES

6.2 In Chapter 2 (paragraph 24), we describe general-purpose external reporting of patient service revenues. The relationship between the records maintained for internal managerial purposes and the general-purpose external reports is discussed in Chapter 3, paragraph 10. For internal accounting purposes, patient service revenues consist of the charges, at the hospital's full established rates, for goods and services provided to patients, regardless of the amounts actually paid to the hospital by or on behalf of patients. The objectives of patient service revenue accounting are to compile (1) a complete and accurate record, on the accrual basis, of revenues classified by revenue centers, by type of patient, by type of payor, and in other useful ways, and (2) a record of revenue deductions, classified by type and in other useful ways. In most cases, the hospital receives less than its established rates, or nothing, for the goods and services provided. It is important to develop quantitative information about revenue "losses" resulting from contractual adjustments, charity services, and other factors resulting in an inability to collect full established rates (see paragraph 6.5).

6.3 Patient service expenses are those that are incurred in providing nursing and other professional services to patients. Expenses are expired costs, that is, costs that have been consumed in carrying on an activity during an accounting period and from which no future measurable benefit is obtained. Expenses represent actual or expected cash outflows (or the equivalent) that have occurred or will eventuate as a result of the entity's ongoing major or central operations. The objective of expense accounting is to accumulate, on an accrual basis, complete and accurate records of expenses in a manner that clearly associates them with the responsibility centers in which the expenses are incurred. Within each center, a secondary classification of expenses should be made according to object of expenditure (natural classification) through the use of the two-digit suffix in the numerical coding system illustrated in Figure 4-3.

6.4 A description of the patient service revenue and expense accounts is provided in Figure 6-1. The indicated account numbers do not include the entity designator, fund designator, or the two-digit suffix discussed in Chapter 4. General departments are identified by the first two digits of the four-digit field; specific departments of the general departments are identified by the last two digits of the four-digit field.

Figure 6-1
Patient Service Revenues and Expenses

Account Numbers

Expenses Revenues

6-0100 **Nursing Services, General**

Some nursing expenses cannot be directly identified with individual nursing units (stations or departments) because they relate to the overall direction of the nursing function or to more than one responsibility center (nursing unit). These expenses may be charged to this account (6-0100) or they may be charged to more specific accounts, such as the following:

Nursing—Administration

Nursing—Staff Development and Education

Nursing—Float Personnel

Nursing—Central Transportation

The activities of some of these specific units are described in the following account descriptions. The expenses incurred by these activities are recorded in the general account (6-0100) if the specific accounts are not used.

6-0110 Nursing—Administration

Nursing administration is responsible for the administration of organized nursing services and the delivery of nursing care to individual patients. This includes all licensed and unlicensed personnel involved in the provision of direct and indirect patient-care activities. Nursing administration includes the scheduling and transferring of nurses between services and units, and nursing staff supervision, evaluation, and discipline.

This responsibility center should be charged with the direct expenses associated with nursing administration. These direct expenses include salaries and wages, professional fees, supplies, and purchased services. Salaries of nurse managers (supervisors) assigned to a single expense center should be charged to that center on a direct assignment basis. The salaries of nurse managers of two or more expense centers

Account Numbers

Expenses Revenues

should be allocated proportionately to those centers. Nurse managers in off-shift supervisor or house supervisor positions should be included in this account (6-0110).

6-0115 Nursing—Staff Development and Education

The hours worked and the salaries paid to nursing personnel while participating in staff development, continuing education, and orientation activities along with other expenses of carrying out all education activities should be charged to this account.

6-0120 Nursing—Float Nursing Personnel

Float nursing personnel includes all nursing personnel in institutional float or per diem programs. It is preferable that the hours worked and the salaries paid to float personnel be charged directly to the departments in which they work. However, these hours and salaries can be initially recorded in this account (6-0120) and then distributed to the appropriate departments on the basis of hours worked. If the latter method is used, all salaries and wages of float personnel must be transferred out of account 6-0120 at the end of each fiscal period. Any idle employee time should be allocated in the same ratio as actual hours worked. After each period's allocation, the balance of account 6-0120 should be zero. Scheduling and other administrative functions relating to float personnel should be included in nursing administration (6-0110). If this specific account (6-0120) is not used, the initial recording of these expenses and their subsequent transfer to the departments in which the work was performed are included in account 6-0100.

6-0125 Nursing—Central Transportation

Central transportation includes the transporting of patients and/or materials between areas in and around the hospital. It does not include the transportation of patients to or from the hospital; these expenses are recorded in account 0-0000. If central transportation is not a nursing function but an activity located in another area of the hospital's organization, the chart of accounts should provide for an account in that area to record the expenses of this activity.

This responsibility center should be charged only with the direct labor expense incurred in operating a central transpor-

Account Numbers

Expenses Revenues

tation service. Account 6-0120 is an interim account only; its balance should be transferred to the appropriate nursing service responsibility center expense accounts at the end of each fiscal period on the basis of hours of service to each center.

6-0200 4-0200 **Nursing Units—Medical and Surgical Acute**

Activities associated with nursing units (stations) of all types may include, but are not limited to: serving and feeding patients; collecting sputum, urine, and feces samples; monitoring vital life signs; preparing equipment and assisting physicians during patient examination and treatment; changing dressings and cleansing wounds and incisions; observing and recording emotional stability of patients; bathing patients and helping them into and out of bed; observing patients for reactions to drugs; administering specified medications; answering patients' call signals; and keeping patients' personal effects in order. Nursing units provide for the delivery of the full range of nursing and patient-care services by licensed and unlicensed nursing personnel and other hospital personnel. Nursing care is defined by the relevant state nurse practice act, applicable regulations, and the hospital's definition of nursing care.

The expenses and revenues associated with nursing units (stations) are properly recorded in specific accounts such as the following:

- Medical and Surgical Acute Care
- Pediatric Acute
- Psychiatric Acute
- Other Adult and Pediatric Acute
- Obstetric (Gynecologic) Acute
- Newborn Nursery Acute

The specific activities of some of these units are indicated in the following descriptions of the major categories of these nursing units.

Account Numbers		
Expenses	**Revenues**	
6–0210 to 6–0490	4–0210 to 4–0490	**Medical and Surgical Acute Care Units**

A hospital usually has many medical and surgical acute care units (stations), which may be identified by location (building, wing, floor), specialization, and/or service. A large number of accounts have been provided here to accommodate the various methods of identification.

Medical and surgical acute care nursing units provide nursing care to individual patients based on professional, hospital, and unit standards of patient care, standards of nursing care, and established protocols and procedures. The general activities of these units are described in account 6-0200.

These responsibility centers should be charged for all direct expenses incurred, and credited with all revenues generated, in providing daily bedside nursing care to medical and surgical patients.

6-0500 4-0500 **Pediatric Acute**

Pediatric acute care units provide nursing care to pediatric patients based on professional, hospital, and unit standards of patient care, standards of nursing care, and established protocol and procedures. The general activities of these units are described in account 6-0200.

These responsibility centers should be charged with all direct expenses incurred, and credited with all revenues generated, in providing daily bedside nursing care to pediatric patients.

6-0600 4-0600 **Psychiatric Acute**

Psychiatric acute care units provide nursing care to patients admitted for diagnosis and/or treatment based on professional, hospital, and unit standards of patient care, standards of nursing care, and established protocol and procedures. The general activities of these units are described in account 6-0200.

These responsibility centers should be charged for all direct expenses incurred, and all revenues generated, in providing daily bedside nursing care to psychiatric patients.

Account Numbers

Expenses Revenues

6-0700 4-0700 **Obstetric (Gynecologic) Acute**

Provision of nursing care to mothers following delivery is provided in the obstetric acute care unit based on professional, hospital, and unit standards of patient care, standards of nursing care, and established protocols and procedures. This unit may also provide care for noninfectious gynecology patients when this practice is allowed by state law and provided for in medical staff rules and regulations. The general activities of this unit are described in account 6-0200.

This responsibility center should be charged with all direct expenses incurred, and credited with all revenues generated, in providing daily bedside nursing care to obstetric (gynecologic) patients.

6-0800 4-0800 **Newborn Nursery Acute**

Daily nursing care for newborn infants is provided in nursery units based on professional, hospital, and unit standards of patient care, standards of nursing care, and established protocols and procedures. The general activities of these units are described in account 6-0200.

Separate accounts for specialized newborn nursery acute care units, such as those listed below, may be maintained. If these separate accounts are used, the general accounts (6-0800 and 4-0800) should not be used.

6-0810 4-0810 Premature Units

Daily nursing care for premature infants is provided in these nursery units based on professional, hospital, and unit standards of patient care, standards of nursing care, and established protocols and procedures. The general activities of these units are described in account 6-0200.

These responsibility centers should be charged with all direct expenses incurred, and credited with all revenues generated, in providing daily bedside nursing care to premature nursery patients. If these separate accounts are not used, the expenses and revenues are recorded in accounts 6-0800 and 4-0800.

Account Numbers		
Expenses	Revenues	
6-0820	4-0820	Normal Delivery Units

Daily nursing care for normal delivery infants is provided in these nursery units based on professional, hospital, and unit standards of patient care, standards of nursing care, and established protocols and procedures. The general activities of these units are described in account 6-0200.

These responsibility centers should be charged with all direct expenses incurred, and credited with all revenues generated, in providing daily bedside nursing care to normal delivery nursery patients. If these specific accounts are not used, the expenses and revenues are recorded in accounts 6-0800 and 4-0800.

6-0900 4-0900 **Other Adult and Pediatric Acute Care Units**

Additional specialized acute care nursing units, such as those listed below, can be established when they are formally organized and staffed inside the hospital. These nursing units provide nursing care to individual patients based on professional, hospital, and unit standards of patient care, Standards of nursing care, and established protocols and procedures. Expenses and revenues relating to these nursing activities can be recorded in general accounts 6-0900 and 4-0900 if the following specific accounts are not used (if the specific accounts are used, these general accounts should not be used).

6-0910 4-0910 Detoxification Unit

Activities of this unit are described in account 6-0900. If these specific accounts are not used, the expenses and revenues related to this unit are recorded in accounts 6-0900 and 4-0900.

6-0920 4-0920 Communicable Disease Unit

Activities of this unit are described in account 6-0900. If these specific accounts are not used, the expenses and revenues related to this unit are recorded in accounts 6-0900 and 4-0900.

6-1200 4-1200 **Intensive Care**

A hospital may have a number of intensive care units such as those described below. Each of these units is staffed with

Account Numbers		
Expenses	Revenues	
		specially trained nursing personnel and contains monitoring and specialized support equipment for treatment of patients who, because of shock, trauma, or other life-threatening conditions, require intensified, comprehensive observation and care. Nursing care is provided to individual patients based on professional, hospital, and unit standards, standards of nursing care, and established protocols and procedures. The activities of these units can be included in general accounts 6-1200 and 4-1200 (if the following specific accounts are used, the general accounts should not be used).
6-1210	4-1210	Medical and Surgical Unit
		A medical/surgical intensive care unit provides patient care of a more intensive nature than that provided to the usual medical, surgical, and pediatric patients. Activities of this unit are described in account 6-1200. If these specific accounts are not used, the expenses and revenues related to this unit are recorded in general accounts 6-1200 and 4-1200.
		These specific accounts should be charged with direct expenses incurred, and credited with all revenues generated, in providing intensive daily bedside nursing care to medical/surgical intensive care patients.
6-1220	4-1220	Pediatric Unit
		A pediatric intensive care unit provides nursing care to pediatric patients that is of a more intensive nature than that usually provided to pediatric patients. Activities of this unit are described in account 6-1200. If these specific accounts are not used, the expenses and revenues related to this unit are recorded in general accounts 6-1200 and 4-1200.
		These specific accounts should be charged with all direct expenses incurred, and credited for all revenues generated, in providing daily bedside nursing care to pediatric intensive care patients.
6-1230	4-1230	Neonatal Unit
		A neonatal intensive care unit provides care to newborn infants that is of a more intensive nature than nursing care provided in newborn acute units. Activities of this unit are described in account 6-1200. If these specific accounts are

Account Numbers		
Expenses	Revenues	
		not used, the expenses and revenues related to this unit are recorded in general accounts 6-1200 and 4-1200. These specific accounts should be charged with all direct expenses incurred, and credited with all revenues generated, in providing daily bedside nursing care to neonatal patients.
6-1240	4-1240	Definitive Observation Unit Definitive-observation intensive care units provide nursing care to patients who are less acutely ill than those requiring admission to medical/surgical intensive care or cardiac care units but who are more acutely ill than those patients requiring admission to a general medical or surgical care unit. Activities of this unit are described in account 6-1200. If these specific accounts are not used, the expenses and revenues related to this unit are recorded in general accounts 6-1200 and 4-1200. These specific accounts should be charged with all direct expenses incurred, and credited with all revenues generated, in providing daily bedside nursing care to definitive observation patients.
6-1250	4-1250	Psychiatric Psychiatric (isolation) intensive care units provide nursing care to psychiatric patients that is of a more intensive nature than the usual nursing care provided in medical, surgical, and psychiatric units. The activities of this unit are described in account 6-1200. If these specific accounts are not used, the expenses and revenues related to this unit are recorded in general accounts 6-1200 and 4-1200. These specific accounts should be charged with all direct expenses incurred, and credited with all revenues generated, in providing daily bedside nursing care to psychiatric patients.
6-1300	4-1300	**Burn Care** A burn care unit provides nursing care to severely burned patients that is of a more intensive nature than the usual acute nursing care provided in medical and surgical units. Burn care units are staffed with specially trained nursing personnel and

Account Numbers		
Expenses	Revenues	
		contain specialized support equipment for burn patients who require intensified, comprehensive observation and care.
		This responsibility center should be charged with all direct expenses incurred, and credited with all revenues generated, in providing daily bedside nursing care to intensive care burn patients.
6-1400	4-1400	**Cardiac Care**
		The delivery of nursing care of a more specialized nature than that usually provided to medical, surgical, and pediatric patients is provided in the cardiac care unit (which can be further organized into specialized units as indicated below). The unit is staffed with specially trained nursing personnel and contains monitoring and specialized support or treatment equipment for patients who, because of heart seizure or other life-threatening conditions, require intensified, comprehensive observation and care. If the following specific accounts are not used, the expenses and revenues related to cardiac care are recorded in general accounts 6-1400 and 4-1400.
6-1410	4-1410	Myocardial Infarction Unit
6-1420	4-1420	Pulmonary Unit
6-1430	4-1430	Heart Transplant Unit
		These responsibility centers should be charged with all direct expenses incurred, and credited with all revenues generated, in providing intensive daily bedside nursing care to cardiac care patients. If these specific accounts are used, the general accounts 6-1400 and 4-1400 should not be used.
6-1500	4-1500	**Extended (Long-Term) and Other Nonacute Care Unit**
		A hospital may have a number of nursing units that provide convalescent, rehabilitative, and/or restorative services at a level less intensive than that of medical, surgical, or pediatric acute care. These services are provided to individual patients based on professional, hospital, and unit standards of patient care, standards of nursing care, and established protocols and procedures. Admissions to these units are usually for periods of 30 days or more.

Account Numbers		
Expenses	Revenues	

The activities of this general unit can be organized into two or more specific units as indicated below. If the specific accounts are not used, all related expenses and revenues should be recorded in general accounts 6-1500 and 4-1500.

These responsibility centers should be charged with all direct expenses incurred, and credited with all revenues generated, in providing daily bedside nursing care to patients requiring extended skilled nursing care usually lasting 30 days or more.

6-1510 4-1510 Skilled Nursing Unit

6-1520 4-1520 Rehabilitation Unit

6-1530 4-1530 Long-Term Psychiatric Unit

Medical care, nursing services, and intensive supervision of chronically mentally ill, mentally disordered, or other mentally incompetent persons are rendered in the long-term psychiatric unit. This responsibility center should be charged with all direct expenses incurred, and credited for all revenues generated, in providing daily bedside nursing care to long-term psychiatric patients.

6-1540 4-1540 Residential Unit

Residential care is the provision of safe, hygienic, sheltered living for residents not capable of fully independent living. Regular and frequent, but not continuous, medical and nursing services are provided. This responsibility center should be charged with all direct expenses incurred, and credited with all revenues generated, in providing nursing care to residential care patients.

6-1550 4-1550 Self-Care Unit

The self-care unit provide supportive, restorative, and preventive health care for ambulatory patients who are capable of caring for themselves under the supervision of a professional nurse. This unit is used by recovering patients who are making the transition to discharge or by patients who are undergoing tests and medical evaluation who require a minimal amount of nursing supervision. These patients generally eat in a central dining facility and do not require bedside nursing care. This responsibility center should be charged with all direct expenses incurred, and credited with all reve-

Account Numbers		
Expenses	Revenues	
		nues generated, in providing nursing care to self-care patients. If this specific account is not used, these expenses and revenues are recorded in general accounts 6-1500 and 4-1500.
6-1600	4-1600	**Hemodialysis**
		Hemodialysis is the purification of the patient's blood through use of an artificial kidney machine or similar device. Additional activities can include, but are not limited to: wheeling portable equipment to patients' bedsides; explaining procedures to patients; operating hemodialysis equipment; and inspecting, testing, and maintaining special equipment. This responsibility center should be charged with all direct expenses incurred, and credited with all revenues generated, in providing hemodialysis services to patients.
6-1700	4-1700	**Respiratory Services**
		All respiratory expenses and revenues can be assigned to these general accounts (6-1700 and 4-1700) or can be assigned to more specific accounts as indicated below. If specific accounts are used, the general accounts should not be used.
6-1710	4-1710	Respiratory Therapy
		Respiratory therapy consists of the administration of oxygen and certain potent drugs through inhalation or positive pressure and provision of other forms of rehabilitative therapy as prescribed by physicians. This function is performed by specially trained personnel who initiate, monitor, and evaluate patient reactions to therapy. This responsibility center should be charged with all direct expenses incurred, and credited with all revenues generated, in providing respiratory therapy services.
6-1720	4-1720	Pulmonary Function Testing
		Pulmonary function testing evaluates patients' ability to exchange oxygen and other gases, through measurement of inhaled and exhaled gases and analysis of blood. This function is performed by specially trained personnel who initiate, monitor, and evaluate patient performance, cooperation, and ability during the testing procedure.

Account Numbers		
Expenses	Revenues	
		This responsibility center should be charged with all direct expenses incurred, and credited with all revenues generated, in providing pulmonary function testing services.
6-1900	4-1900	**Labor and Delivery Services**
		Included in this responsibility center are the labor and delivery services provided by specially trained nursing personnel to patients, including prenatal care during labor, assistance during delivery, postnatal care in the recovery room, and minor gynecologic procedures if they are performed in the delivery suite.
		All labor and delivery services expenses and revenues can be assigned to general accounts 6-1900 and 4-1900, or can be assigned to more specific accounts as indicated below. If these specific accounts are used, the general accounts should not be used.
6-1910	4-1910	Labor Rooms
6-1920	4-1920	Delivery Rooms
		These responsibility centers should be charged with all direct expenses incurred, and credited with all revenues generated, in providing labor and delivery services to patients.
6-2100	4-2100	**Surgical Services**
		Surgical services are provided to patients by specially trained nursing personnel who assist physicians in the performance of surgical and related procedures during and immediately following surgery.
		All of the surgical services expenses and revenues may be assigned to general accounts 6-2100 and 4-2100, or can be assigned to more specific accounts as indicated below. If specific accounts are used, the general accounts should not be used.
6-2101		Administrative Office
6-2110	4-2110	General Surgery
6-2120	4-2120	Organ Transplants
6-2130	4-2130	Open-Heart Surgery

Account Numbers		
Expenses	Revenues	
6-2140	4-2140	Neurosurgery
6-2150	4-2150	Orthopedic Surgery
6-2160	4-2160	Minor Surgery
6-2170	4-2170	Surgical Day Care (Minisurgery)
6-2180	4-2180	Recovery Rooms

These responsibility centers should be charged with all direct expenses incurred, and credited with all revenues generated, in providing surgical services to patients.

6-2300 4-2300 **Emergency and Ambulance Services**

Hospitals usually provide emergency medical care and ambulance services to patients. All associated expenses and revenues may be assigned to general accounts 6-2300 and 4-2300, or can be assigned to more specific accounts as indicated below. If the specific accounts are used, the general accounts should not be used.

6-2310 4-2310 Emergency Department

This responsibility center provides emergency treatment, usually on an unscheduled basis, to the ill and injured who require immediate medical or surgical care. These activities are classified as outpatient services, but expense and revenue amounts related to patients who are admitted as inpatients may be transferred to the nursing units to which the patients are admitted. Additional activities can include, but are not limited to: comforting patients; maintaining aseptic conditions; assisting physicians in performance of emergency care; monitoring vital life signs; applying bandages or assisting physicians in applying bandages; coordinating the scheduling of patients through required professional service functions; and completing patient records.

This responsibility center should be charged with all direct expenses incurred, and credited with all revenues generated, in providing emergency treatment to the ill and injured.

6-2315 4-2315 Ambulance Service

This responsibility center provides ambulance service, usually on an unscheduled basis, to the ill and injured who require

Account Numbers		
Expenses	Revenues	
		immediate medical attention. Additional activities can include, but are not limited to: lifting patients into and out of an ambulance; transporting patients to and from the hospital; and providing first-aid treatment administered by a physician or a physician's assistant prior to arrival at the hospital.
		This responsibility center should be charged with all direct expenses incurred, and credited with all revenues generated, in providing ambulance service to the ill and injured.
6-2320	4-2320	**Private Referred Ambulatory**
		This department provides registration for private referred ambulatory patients who require diagnostic testing or other services from ancillary departments such as laboratory or radiology. In some cases, the private referred ambulatory department may provide direct patient services. These patients have been referred by a physician for the services they obtain.
		This responsibility center should be charged with all direct expenses incurred in the registration of private ambulatory patients. Revenues would only be generated if this center provided the ancillary services, and the direct expenses of providing those services should be charged to this center.
6-2500	4-2500	**Central Services and Sterile Supply**
		The central services and sterile supply function is to prepare and issue medical and surgical supplies and equipment to patients and to hospital expense centers. Other activities can include, but are not limited to: requisitioning and issuing appropriate supply items that are required for patient care; preparing sterile irrigating solutions; collecting, assembling, sterilizing, and redistributing reusable items; and cleaning, assembling, maintaining, and issuing portable apparatus.
		All direct expenses incurred and all revenues generated in preparing and issuing medical and surgical supplies and equipment to patients can be assigned to general accounts 6-2500 and 4-2500, or can be assigned to more specific accounts as indicated below. If the specific accounts are used, the general accounts should not be used.

Account Numbers		
Expenses	**Revenues**	
6-2510	4-2510	Central Services
6-2520	4-2520	Central Sterile Supply

Appropriate object codes (using the two-digit suffix illustrated in Chapter 4) should be established to accumulate expenses of these centers under the natural classification system. The invoice cost of supplies and equipment that are not billed to patients and are issued to other responsibility centers should be transferred to the accounts of the consuming responsibility centers on a periodic basis. If a central materials management department combining the functions of purchasing, stores, and central services and supply is maintained, the expenses of that department should be reclassified to central services and supplies and to the purchasing department on a periodic basis.

6-3100 4-3100 **Laboratory Services**

The laboratory services function is to perform diagnostic and routine laboratory tests, including maintenance of equipment and quality control standards, transportation of specimens from nursing floors and operating rooms, and preparation of samples for testing. All laboratory service expense and revenue can be assigned to general accounts 6-3100 and 4-3100, or can be assigned to more specific accounts such as the following (if the specific accounts are used, the general accounts should not be used):

Expenses	Revenues	
6-3110		Administrative Office
6-3115		Animal Maintenance
6-3120	4-3120	Autopsy
6-3125	4-3125	Blood Bank (described below)
6-3130	4-3130	Chemistry
6-3135	4-3135	Hematology
6-3140	4-3140	Histology (mortuary operations may be included or recorded in a separate responsibility center)
6-3145	4-3145	Immunology
6-3150	4-3150	Microbiology

Account Numbers		
Expenses	**Revenues**	
6-3155		Procurement and Dispatch
6-3160	4-3160	Radioisotopes
6-3165	4-3165	Special Procedures
6-3170	4-3170	Urine and Feces

The blood bank procures, receives, and stores a supply of whole blood and blood derivatives. Additional activities can include, but are not limited to: processing and issuing whole blood derivatives; producing blood derivatives from whole blood; and recruiting donors and collecting blood.

This responsibility center should be charged with all direct expenses incurred, and credited with all revenues generated, in maintaining a separate blood bank within the hospital. The two-digit suffix should be used to provide for a secondary classification of the revenues and expenses of this center as illustrated in Figures 4-2 and 4-3.

When blood is purchased, its cost (including Red Cross and similar administrative fees) is the amount paid. When blood is donated, its cost is its fair market value at date of donation, and an offsetting credit is made to Donated Commodities, account 5-4120. The cost of blood (amount paid for it or its fair market value) is charged to blood bank expense, or to an inventory account, if applicable. This cost is not debited to revenue or cleared through an agency account.

6-3300 4-3300 **Electrodiagnosis**

This department operates specialized equipment that records electromotive variations in the movements of the heart on an electrocardiograph to facilitate diagnosis of heart disease. Additional activities can include, but are not limited to: wheeling portable equipment to patients' bedsides; explaining test procedures to patients; operating electrocardiograph equipment; inspecting, testing, and maintaining special equipment; and attaching electrodes to and removing them from patients. All electrodiagnosis expenses and revenues can be assigned to general accounts 6-3300 and 4-3300 or can be assigned to more specific accounts, such as the following (if specific accounts are used, the general accounts should not be used):

Account Numbers		
Expenses	Revenues	
6-3310		Administrative Office
6-3320	4-3320	Electrocardiology

Account Numbers

Expenses Revenues

6-3310 Administrative Office

This account is used to record all expenses related to the maintenance of an electrodiagnosis administrative office.

6-3320 4-3320 Electrocardiology

The specialized equipment operated by this responsibility center records electromotive variations in the movements of the heart on an electrocardiograph to facilitate diagnosis of heart disease.

This responsibility center should be charged with all direct expenses incurred, and credited with all revenues generated, in providing electrocardiolgy services to patients.

6-3330 4-3330 Electromyography

This department operates specialized equipment that records electrical potential variations in muscles on an electromyograph to facilitate diagnosis of muscular and nervous disorders.

Additional activities can include, but are not limited to: wheeling portable equipment to patients' bedsides; explaining test procedures to patients; operating electromyograph equipment; inspecting, testing, and maintaining special equipment; and attaching electrodes to and removing them from patients.

This responsibility center should be charged with all direct expenses incurred, and credited with all revenues generated, in providing electromyographic services.

6-3340 4-3340 Electroencephalography

This department operates specialized equipment that records electromotive variations in brain waves on an electroencephalograph for use in diagnosis. This responsibility center should be charged with all direct expenses incurred, and credited with all revenues generated, in performing electroencephalographic services.

6-3400 4-3400 **Radiology—Diagnostic**

Account Numbers

Expenses Revenues

All expenses and revenues related to the provision of diagnostic radiology services can be assigned to general accounts 6-3400 and 4-3400, or can be assigned to more specific accounts such as the following (if specific accounts are used, the general accounts should not be used):

6-3410 Administrative Office

This account is used to record all expenses associated with the maintenance of an administrative office for diagnostic radiology services.

6-3420 4-3420 Angiocardiography

This department provides diagnostic radiology services under the direction of a qualified radiologist as required for the examination and care of patients. Diagnostic radiology services include taking, processing, examining, and interpreting radiographs and fluorographs. Additional activities can include, but are not limited to: consultation with patients and attending physicians, radioactive waste disposal, and storage of radioactive materials.

This responsibility center should be charged with all direct expenses incurred, and credited with all revenues generated, in providing diagnostic radiology services to patients.

6-3500 4-3500 **Radiology—Therapeutic**

This department provides therapeutic radiology services to patients. All related expenses and revenues can be assigned to general accounts 6-3500 and 4-3500, or can be assigned to more specific accounts as follows (if specific accounts are used, the general accounts are not used):

6-3510 Administrative Office

All expenses related to the maintenance of a therapeutic radiology administrative office are charged to this account.

6-3520 4-3520 Medical Oncology (Chemotherapy)

This department provides medical treatment for patients with malignant or hematologic disorders. Patients are seen by certified medical oncologists for initial and recurring visits. Patients may undergo various diagnostic procedures such as bone marrow aspiration or receive treatments including, but

Account Numbers		
Expenses	Revenues	

not limited to, chemotherapy, blood product administration, antibiotic administration, and/or treatments with biologic response modifiers. Symptom management related to the disease or treatment is also provided. Additional services can include initial and comprehensive assessments, consultation, and education.

This responsibility center should be charged with all direct expenses incurred, and credited with all revenues generated, in the provision of medical oncology services to patients.

6-3530 4-3530 Radiation Therapy

This department provides therapeutic radiology services under the direction of a qualified radiologist as required for the care and treatment of patients. Therapeutic radiology services include therapy using radium and radioactive substances. Additional activities can include, but are not limited to: consultation with patients and attending physicians, radioactive waste disposal, and storage of radioactive materials.

This responsibility center should be charged with all direct expenses incurred, and credited with all revenues generated, in providing therapeutic radiology services.

6-3600 4-3600 **Nuclear Medicine**

This department provides diagnosis and treatment under the direction of a qualified physician through use of injectable or ingestible radioactive isotopes as required for the care and treatment of patients. Additional activities can include, but are not limited to: consultation with patients and attending physicians, radioactive waste disposal, and storage of radioactive materials.

All expenses and revenues related to the provision of nuclear medicine services can be assigned to general accounts 6-3600 and 4-3600, or can be assigned to more specific accounts such as the following (if specific accounts are used, the general accounts should not be used):

6-3610 Administrative Office

This account is used to record all expenses related to the maintenance of a nuclear medicine administrative office.

Account Numbers

Expenses	Revenues	
6-3620	4-3620	Nuclear Medicine—Diagnostic

This department provides diagnosis under the direction of a qualified physician through the use of injectable and/or ingestible radioactive pharmaceuticals as required for the care and treatment of patients. Additional activities can include, but are not limited to: consultation with patients and attending physicians, radioactive waste disposal, and the receiving and storage of radioactive materials.

This responsibility center should be charged with all direct expenses incurred, and credited with all revenues generated, in providing diagnostic nuclear medicine services to patients.

6-3630 4-3630 Nuclear Medicine—Therapeutic

This department provides therapeutic nuclear medicine services under the direction of a qualified physician through the use of ingestible radioactive pharmaceuticals as required for the care and treatment of patients. Additional activities can include, but are not limited to: consultation with patients and attending physicians, radioactive waste disposal, the receiving and storage of radioactive materials, and radioactive decontamination.

This responsibility center should be charged with all direct expenses incurred, and credited with all revenues generated, in providing therapeutic nuclear medicine services to patients.

6-3700 4-3700 **Pharmacy**

This department produces, preserves, stores, compounds, manufactures, packages, controls, assays, dispenses, and distributes medications (including intravenous solutions) for inpatients and outpatients under the direction of a licensed pharmacist. Pharmacy services include the maintenance in designated areas of separate stocks of commonly used items.

Additional activities can include, but are not limited to: development and maintenance of formularies established by the medical staff, consultation with and advice to medical and nursing staff on drug therapy, adding drugs to intravenous solutions, determining incompatibility in drug combinations, and stocking floor drugs and dispensing machines.

Account Numbers		
Expenses	**Revenues**	
		This responsibility center should be charged with all direct expenses incurred, and credited with all revenues generated, in maintaining a pharmacy under the direction of a licensed pharmacist. Appropriate use should be made of the two-digit suffix to provide for a natural (object of expenditure) classification of the expenses of this center. The cost of supplies that are not billed to patients and are issued at invoice cost to other responsibility centers should be transferred to the accounts of the consuming responsibility centers on a periodic basis.
6-3800	4-3800	**Anesthesiology**
		Anesthesia services are rendered in the hospital by, or under the direction of, a physician trained in anesthesia or the operating surgeon. Additional activities can include, but are not limited to: recording type and amount of anesthetic administered; conducting physical examinations of patients; observing patient's condition until all effects of the anesthesia have passed; obtaining laboratory findings before anesthetic is administered; administering treatment to patients having symptoms of postanesthesia complications; accompanying patients to recovery room or intensive care units; prescribing preanesthesia and postanesthesia medications; and establishing and carrying out safeguards for administration of anesthetics.
		This responsibility center should be charged with all direct expenses incurred, and credited with all revenues generated, in administering anesthetics under the direction of a physician.
6-3900	4-3900	**Rehabilitation Services**
		All expenses and revenues related to the provision of rehabilitation services can be assigned to general accounts 6-3900 and 4-3900, or can be assigned to more specific accounts such as the following (if specific accounts are used, the general accounts should not be used):
6-3910		Administrative Office
		This account is used to record all expenses related to the maintenance of an administrative office for rehabilitation services.

Account Numbers

Expenses Revenues

6-3920 4-3920 Physical Therapy

The physical therapy department employs therapeutic exercises and massage and utilizes effective properties of light, heat, cold, water, and electricity for diagnosis and rehabilitation of patients who have neuromuscular, orthopedic, and other disabilities. These services are provided under the direction of a physician or registered physical therapist. Physical therapy services include the provision of clinical and consultative services and the direction of patients in the use, function, and care of braces, artificial limbs, and other devices. Additional activities can include, but are not limited to: prescribing therapeutic exercises; counseling patients and their relatives; organizing and conducting medically prescribed physical therapy programs; applying diagnostic muscle tests; administering whirlpool and compact baths; changing linen on beds and treatment tables; and assisting patients in changing clothes.

This responsibility center should be charged with all direct expenses incurred, and credited with all revenues generated, in maintaining a physical therapy program.

6-3930 4-3930 Occupational Therapy

Occupational therapy includes teaching manual skills and independence in personal care to stimulate mental and emotional activity on the part of patients. Services include instructing patients in prescribed academic subjects to prevent mental deconditioning, improving patients' mental and physical conditions, and aiding in the attainment of knowledge and skills that will further patients' progress toward vocational objectives. Additional activities can include, but are not limited to: counseling patients' relatives and employers on both individual case and group bases, administering accreditation and other academic tests, and instructing patients in technical aspects of work.

This responsibility center should be charged with all direct expenses incurred, and credited with all revenues generated, in maintaining an occupational therapy program.

6-3940 4-3940 Speech Therapy

Speech therapy encompasses the evaluation and treatment of persons with communication and/or swallowing problems.

Account Numbers

Expenses	Revenues	

Specifically, rehabilitation of communication skills includes the areas of speech, voice, fluency, and language. Deficiencies in these areas may result from stroke, head injury, cancer, and other causes. Patients are seen by a licensed speech/language pathologist holding a masters' degree from an accredited university program. Services included are assessment, treatment, and counseling patients in their deficit areas, and involves the use of oral, vocal and speech exercises, augmentative/alternative communication, and language stimulation activities to address specific weaknesses. Compensatory strategies and assistive devices are used to maximize communication potentials. In the specialized area of swallowing, videofluoroscopies are employed to assist in diagnosing and determining the nature of the swallowing disorder as well as planning treatment strategies. Additional activities can include, but are not limited to, counseling patients' families and designing treatment programs.

This responsibility center should be charged with all direct expenses incurred, and credited with all revenues generated, in providing speech therapy services to patients.

6-3950 4-3950 Recreational Therapy

Recreational therapy is the process of using recreation/leisure activities as a tool in patient evaluation and treatment, addressing the physical, cognitive, and social aspects of a person, and developing a plan to re-integrate the patient back into the community. The services are provided by personnel who are qualified by education, training, and experience. Additional activities can include, but are not limited to: leisure planning, community re-entry outings, competitive sports for the disabled, and general endurance training.

This responsibility center should be charged with all direct expenses incurred, and credited with all revenues generated, in the provision of recreational therapy services to patients.

6-4100 4-4100 **Clinic Services**

Clinics provide organized diagnostic, preventive, curative, rehabilitative, and educational services on a scheduled basis to ambulatory patients. Additional activities can include, but are not limited to: participating in community activities designed to promote health education; diagnosing and treating ambulatory patients who have illnesses that respond quickly

Account Numbers		
Expenses	Revenues	
		to treatment; referring patients who require prolonged or specialized care to appropriate other services; assigning patients to physicians in accordance with clinic rules; assisting and guiding volunteers in their duties; and making patients' appointments through required professional service functions.
		All expenses and revenues related to clinic services can be assigned to general accounts 6-4100 and 4-4100, or can be recorded in more specific accounts such as the following (if specific accounts are used, the general accounts should not be used):
6-4110		Administrative Office
6-4115	4-4115	Cardiology Clinic
6-4120	4-4120	Eye, Ear, Nose, and Throat Clinic
6-4125	4-4125	Medical and Surgical Clinic
6-4130	4-4130	Obstetrics and Gynecology Clinic
6-4135	4-4135	Orthopedics Clinic
6-4140	4-4140	Pediatrics Clinic
6-4145	4-4145	Physical Medicine Clinic
6-4150	4-4150	Psychiatric Clinic
6-4155	4-4155	Urology Clinic
6-4300	4-4300	**Home Care**
		Home care encompasses a broad spectrum of both health and social services that can be delivered to the recovering, disabled, or chronically ill person in the home environment. These services include the traditional core of professional nursing and home care aide services as well as physical therapy, occupational therapy, speech therapy, medical social services, and nutritional services. Hospice is a special component of home care involving medical, social, psychological, and spiritual care for terminally ill patients and their families. It is aimed at relieving pain and suffering and providing the most comfortable environment possible, allowing a terminally ill person to die with dignity.

Account Numbers		
Expenses	Revenues	
		All expenses and revenues related to the provision of home care services can be assigned to general accounts 6-4300 and 4-4300, or can be assigned to more specific accounts such as the following (if specific accounts are used, the general accounts are not used):
6-4310		Administrative Office
6-4320	4-4320	Hospice
6-4330	4-4330	Nursing Service
6-4340	4-4340	Rehabilitation Service
		Home health services provide nursing care to patients at their places of residence. Activities involved in each of the following functions can be performed for patients outside the hospital: nursing care, physical therapy, intravenous therapy, inhalation therapy, electrocardiology, occupational and recreational therapy, social service, dietary, and housekeeping.
6-4400	4-4400	**Social Services**
		The social service department obtains, analyzes, and interprets social and economic information about patients that aids in diagnosis, treatment, and rehabilitation. This service includes counseling staff and patients in case units and group units and participating in development of community social and health education programs. Additional activities can include, but are not limited to: interviewing patients and relatives to obtain social history relevant to medical problems and planning; interpreting problems of social situations as they relate to medical conditions and/or hospitalization; arranging for postdischarge care of the chronically ill; and collecting and revising information on community health and welfare resources.
		This responsibility center should be charged for all direct expenses incurred, and credited for all revenues generated, in providing social services to patients.
6-4500		**Health Records and Library Services**
6-4510		Health Records
		The health (medical) records department creates and utilizes systems and standards to ensure the collection, transcription,

Account Numbers

Expenses Revenues

storage, destruction, and release of quality health information. The department manages patient privacy through controlled release of information policies and assigns codes for reimbursement. The department produces and maintains indexes, abstracts, and statistical data including daily census to support hospital programs. Analysis and tracking systems (manual or computerized) of health records are established and maintained by this department. In some hospitals, the department may manage registries (including tumor, medical device, and birth registries) and collect data for completion of birth certificates.

Expenses associated with storage, destruction, and microfilming of patient health records should be charged to this department. Fees derived from requests for health records and abstracts should be credited to account 5-3500.

6-4520 Medical Library

The medical library procures, stores, indexes, classifies, annotates, and abstracts books, catalogs, journals, and other related published materials, principally for medical staff use. It also reviews library records for completeness and compliance with established standards.

This responsibility center should be charged with all direct expenses incurred in maintaining the medical library function.

DEDUCTIONS FROM REVENUES

6.5 The deductions from revenues accounts are used only for purposes of internal accounting. In external general-purpose financial statements, the amount to be reported as patient service revenues is the total dollar amount recorded in the 4-0000 series of accounts minus the total dollar amount recorded in the 5-1000 series of accounts. Bad debts are not recorded or reported as deductions from revenues; bad debts are recorded and reported as expenses of the credits and collections department (see account 7-7310). The recording and reporting of bad debts are discussed in Chapter 3, paragraph 11.

6.6 Accounts used in internal accounting for deductions from revenues are described in Figure 6-2. Account numbers are presented under the "expenses" column because deductions from revenues accounts have debit balances. These accounts are contrarevenue accounts.

Figure 6-2
Deductions from Revenues

Account Numbers

Expenses Revenues

5-1100 **Contractual Adjustments**

5-1110 Medicare Standard Arrangement

5-1120 Public Aid Programs

5-1130 Charge-Based Third Parties

5-1140 Third-Party Risk Arrangements

5-1150 Other Third Parties

These accounts are charged with the differential (if any) between the amount, based on the hospital's full established rates, of charges to patients for services rendered during the period, and the amounts received or due from third-party payers in payment for such services. Offsetting credits are made to the appropriate allowance for uncollectible receivables account (1-3320).

5-1200 **Charity Services**

5-1210 Charity Services—Inpatients

This account should be charged with the periodic estimates of the amounts of inpatient accounts receivable that are likely to be uncollectible because the patient met the hospital's charity service criteria at the time of service. The off-setting credit is made to account 1-331, Allowance for Uncollectible Receivables—Inpatient Charity Services. Accounting for, and financial reporting of, charity service is described in Chapter 3, paragraphs 10 through 13. The estimated amount of charity services can be based on a percentage applied to the balances of inpatient receivables or the amount of charges made to inpatients' accounts during a given period, or it can be based on a detailed analysis (aging schedule) of inpatient accounts.

Each hospital must establish its own criteria for distinguishing between uncollectible accounts that should be considered charity write-offs and those that should be considered bad debts. Bad debts result from a failure to make payment even

Account Numbers

Expenses Revenues

though the responsible party has the financial ability to pay. Charity services result from the responsible party fulfilling the criteria established by the hospital.

The criteria may consider factors such as income, net worth, employment status, family size, financial obligations, health-care service needs, and other sources of payment. Because many factors must be considered, judgment is essential, rigid criteria are undesirable, and different hospitals may apply similar criteria differently.

Application of the criteria must consider availability and verification of information. Eligibility for charity service should be determined as soon as possible, even before admission, but it is not necessary that there be a rigid limit on the time when the determination of eligibility for charity service is made. Collection effort is an appropriate part of the process of gathering information about eligibility. Once an amount is determined to qualify as charity services, the amount should be reclassified as bad debts only if the information on which the determination was based is found to be in error. Only the portion of services for which the patient is financially responsible, and is unable to pay, is classified as charity services.

5-1220 Charity Services—Outpatients

This account should be charged with the periodic estimates of the amounts of outpatient accounts receivable that are likely to be uncollectible because the patient met the hospital's charity service criteria at the time of service. The offsetting credit is made to account 1-3332, Allowance for Uncollectible Accounts—Outpatient Charity Services. Account 5-1210 provides additional information about charity services, such as criteria and timing of determination.

5-1300 **Other Revenue Deductions**

5-1310 Courtesy Discounts

5-1320 Administrative Adjustments

Reductions, such as courtesy allowances and employee discounts, from the hospital's established rates for services rendered should be charged to courtesy discounts (account 5-1310) and credited to the appropriate allowance for uncollectible receivables account (account 1-3340).

Account Numbers

Expenses Revenues

The administrative adjustments account (5-1320) is charged or credited for write-offs of immaterial debit or credit balances in patients' accounts in which the cost of billing or refunding exceeds the amount of the account balance.

OTHER REVENUES

6.7 In addition to patient service revenues, a hospital may have several types of revenues and operating gains arising from activities other than patient services that are a part of the hospital's ongoing or central operations (as defined by the individual hospital). The accounts for these other revenues and operating gains are described in Figure 6-3. Refer to Chapter 2, paragraphs 23 and 26 for a discussion of the difference between revenues and gains and the difference between operating gains and nonoperating gains.

Figure 6-3
Other Revenues and Operating Gains

Account Numbers

Expenses Revenues

5-2200 **Tuition**

5-2210 School of Nursing

5-2220 Licensed Vocational Nurse Program

5-2230 Paramedical Education

5-2240 Interns

5-2250 Residents

These accounts are used to record revenues from the school of nursing, licensed vocational nurse program, paramedical, medical postgraduate, and other educational activities.

5-3000 **Cafeteria**

This account is credited for revenues earned in the hospital cafeteria for meals served to employees, visitors, and others. Also included in this account are revenues for meals on wheels, guest meals, and employee catering. Revenues from food-vending machines are included in this account when the cost of the food in these machines is charged to the dietary department.

5-3100 **Laundry and Linen Services**

This account should be credited for revenues earned by providing laundry and linen services to employees and students.

5-3200 **Communication Services**

Amounts received from patients, employees, and others in payment for hospital telephone, fax, and telegram services should be credited to this account.

5-3300 **Parking**

Account Numbers

Expenses Revenues

Amounts received from visitors, employees, and others in payment for parking privileges should be credited to this account.

5-3400 **Television and Radio Rentals**

This account is used to record revenues from television and radio rentals when the activity is hospital-conducted.

5-3500 **Health (Medical) Record and Abstract Fees**

This account is credited for medical record transcript and abstract fees.

5-3600 **Sales of Scrap and Waste**

This account is used to record revenues from sales of miscellaneous scrap and waste.

5-3700 **Vending Machine Commissions**

Commissions earned from coin-operated vending machines and telephones are credited to this account.

5-4000 **Rentals**

5-4010 Student Housing

5-4020 Employee Housing

5-4030 Nonpatient Rooms

5-4040 Physicians' Offices

These accounts are used to record revenues from the rental of housing to students and employees, nonpatients (cots, for example), physicians, and others.

5-4100 **Donated Services and Commodities**

5-4110 Donated Services

5-4120 Donated Commodities

Account Numbers

Expenses Revenues

These accounts are used to record the fair value of services and commodities donated to the hospital. As indicated in Chapter 3, paragraph 28, guidelines exist as to whether donated services should be recorded. If the criteria are met, the fair value of donated services generally should be recorded as other revenues (rather than nonoperating gains).

5-4200 **Cash Discounts, Rebates, and Refunds**

The cost of items purchased generally should be recorded net of discounts, and rebates and refunds should be credited to the account in which the cost was initially recorded. In some cases, however, discounts, rebates, and refunds cannot be attributed to specific purchases, e.g., a rebate from a group purchasing contract that is based on aggregate purchases over a period of time. Discounts, rebates, and refunds that cannot be attributed to specific purchases are recorded in this account (5-1400).

5-5000 **Services to Other Entities**

5-5010 Purchasing

5-5020 Janitorial

5-5030 Laundry and Linen

5-5040 Education

5-5050 Management

5-5060 Data Processing

5-5070 Research Fees and Royalties

These accounts are credited for revenues earned from the provision of the indicated services to other organizations.

5-6000 **Grants and Tax Appropriations**

5-6100 Grants

5-6200 Tax Appropriations

These accounts are used to record revenues received in the form of general-purpose grants and tax appropriations (subsidies).

Account Numbers

Expenses Revenues

5-9000 **Assets Released from Restrictions**

When donor-restricted assets are released from donor restrictions, the amounts of such assets are reclassified from restricted to unrestricted, and the same amounts are reclassified from restricted equity to unrestricted equity. Assets released from restrictions are credited to this account and are reported in the statement of income and other changes in unrestricted equity as shown in Figure 7-2. The following specific accounts may be employed:

5-9100 Satisfaction of Specific Purpose Restrictions

5-9200 Satisfaction of Equipment Acquisition Restrictions

5-9300 Satisfaction of Time Restrictions

GENERAL, FISCAL, AND ADMINISTRATIVE SERVICES EXPENSES

6.8 The responsibility center accounts used to record the expenses incurred in providing general, fiscal, and administrative services are described in Figure 6-4. Within each center, a secondary classification of expenses should be maintained according to object of expenditure (natural classification) through the use of the two-digit suffix as illustrated in Figure 4-3.

Figure 6-4
General, Fiscal, and Administrative Services Expenses

Account Numbers

Expenses Revenues

7-6000 **Dietary Service**

The work of the dietary service includes the procurement, storage, processing, and delivery of food and nourishments to patients and to the cafeteria in compliance with public health regulations and physicians' orders. Additional activities can include, but are not limited to: teaching patients and their families about nutrition and modified diet requirements; determining patient food preferences in terms of type of food and method of preparation; preparing selective menus for various specific diet requirements; preparing or recommending a diet manual, approved by the medical staff, for use by physicians and nurses; and delivering and collecting food trays for meals and nourishments.

This general account can be charged with the direct expenses incurred in preparing, delivering, and collecting food trays for meals and nourishments, and the direct expenses incurred in preparing and delivering food (including formula for infants) to patients and to the cafeteria. Dietary expenses typically are accumulated in more specific accounts such as the following:

7-6010 Administrative Office

This account is used to record the expenses of maintaining an administrative office for the dietary function.

7-6020 Kitchen

This account is used to record expenses that relate to both patient food service and the cafeteria, such as those incurred in procuring, storing, processing, and delivering food and nourishments to patients, employees, and visitors.

This expense center account is charged with all food preparation expenses that are not directly associated with dietary or cafeteria functions. Examples include common salaries of cooks, common food costs, common minor equipment costs, common administrative costs, and so forth. These common costs should be accumulated in this expense center account

Account Numbers

Expenses Revenues

and distributed (preferably on a monthly basis) to the dietary service (account 7-6000) and cafeteria (account 7-6040) expense centers, based on the ratio of number of meals served in each area.

The patient meal count should be made by counting one meal for each tray sent to a patient at mealtime. Nourishments, tube feedings, and infant formulas should be excluded. An equivalent meal count should be made in the cafeteria by use of the following procedures: count a free meal served as a full meal. A full meal consists of meat, potato, vegetable, salad, beverage, and dessert. When there is a selection of entrees, desserts, and so forth at different prices, use an average in calculating the selling price of a full meal. An equivalent meal in a pay cafeteria is determined by dividing total sales by the average selling price of a full meal served at noon.

7-6030 Patient Food Service

The work of the patient food service includes the procurement, storage, processing, and delivery of food and nourishments to patients in compliance with public health regulations and physicians' orders. Additional activities can include, but are not limited to: teaching patients and their families about nutrition and modified diet requirements; determining patient food preferences in terms of type of food and method of preparation; preparing selective menus for various specific diet requirements; preparing or recommending a diet manual, approved by the medical staff, for use by physicians and nurses; and delivering and collecting food trays for meals and nourishments.

This expense center should be charged with all the direct expenses incurred in preparing and delivering food to patients (including infants).

7-6040 Cafeteria

The work of the cafeteria includes the procurement, storage, processing, and delivery of food to employees and to other nonpatients in compliance with public health regulations. This expense center is charged with all expenses directly identifiable with preparing food and serving it to employees and other nonpatients.

Account Numbers

Expenses Revenues

7-6100 **Plant Operation**

Plant operation includes the maintenance and service of utilities such as heat, light, water, air conditioning, and air treatment. Additional activities include, but are not limited to: trash disposal; boiler operation and maintenance; and service and maintenance of water treatment facilities, drainage systems, and utility transmission systems, including such maintenance performed under contract.

The direct expenses incurred in plant operation typically are accumulated in specific responsibility center accounts such as the following:

7-6110 Administrative Office

This expense center should be charged with all direct expenses incurred in maintaining an administrative office for plant operation.

7-6120 Grounds

The grounds department is responsible for maintaining the grounds of the hospital, including landscaped and paved areas, streets on the property, sidewalks, fenced areas and fencing, external recreation areas, and parking facilities.

This expense center account should be charged with all direct expenses incurred in maintaining the grounds of the hospital. This category of maintenance is separated from other activities because its costs have no specific relationship to the size of the hospital or activities performed within it.

7-6130 Boiler and Power Plant

7-6140 Parking

The parking service provides parking facilities to patients, employees, and visitors. This expense center account should be charged with the direct expenses incurred in providing parking facilities owned and/or operated by the hospital. Revenues from parking facilities should not be credited to this expense center account but to other revenues (account 5-3300).

Account Numbers

Expenses	Revenues	
7-6150		Elevator Operation
7-6160		Security

The security department maintains the safety and well-being of hospital patients and personnel, and protects the hospital's facilities. This expense center account should be charged with the direct expenses incurred by the security department in maintaining the safety and well-being of hospital patients, employees, and visitors.

7-6200 **Plant Maintenance**

Plant maintenance includes the maintenance and repair of buildings, parking facilities, and all equipment; painting; elevator maintenance; vehicle maintenance; and performance of minor renovation of buildings and equipment. Additional activities can include, but are not limited to technical assistance on equipment purchases and installation, coordinating construction, and establishing priorities for repairs and utility projects.

A work order system should be developed so that accurate determinations of repair and maintenance costs that are applicable to specific departments are possible. The costs of equipment maintenance and repair that can be directly identified with specific expense centers (for example, the cost to repair x-ray equipment) should be transferred to those specific expense center accounts as preliminary allocations prior to year-end cost finding. Records should be kept to ensure that routine preventive maintenance is performed and to aid in determining when replacement of equipment is more economical than continuing to maintain it.

The direct expenses of plant maintenance can be charged to this general account, or can be charged to more specific accounts, such as those indicated below:

7-6210		Administrative Office
7-6220		Carpentry
7-6230		Plumbing

Account Numbers

Expenses Revenues

7-6240 Painting

7-6250 Electrical and Refrigeration

7-6260 Automotive

7-6300 **Housekeeping Service**

This department is responsible for the care and cleaning of the interior physical plant, including the care (washing, waxing, and stripping) of floors, walls, ceilings, partitions, and windows (inside and outside). Also included are furniture stripping, disinfecting and making beds, care of fixtures (excluding equipment) and furnishings, and emptying room trash containers. This expense center also should be charged with the costs of similar services purchased from outside organizations.

This expense center account should be charged with the direct expenses incurred by the unit responsible for maintaining general cleanliness and sanitation throughout the hospital and other areas (such as student and employee quarters).

7-6400 **Laundry and Linen Services**

The laundry and linen services store, issue, mend, wash, and process in-service linens. The services include work on uniforms, special linens, and disposable linen substitutes.

This general expense center should be charged with the direct expenses incurred in providing laundry and linen services for hospital use, including student and employee quarters. The cost of disposable linen should be recorded in this expense center account.

If desired, laundry and linen service expenses can be accumulated in more specific expense center accounts such as the following:

7-6410 Laundry Service

7-6420 Linen Service

If these specific accounts are used, the general account (7-6400) is not used.

Account Numbers		
Expenses	Revenues	
		FISCAL SERVICES EXPENSES
7-7000		**Fiscal Services**
		The fiscal services function includes accounting, financial management, and related activities. The expenses incurred in carrying out these activities typically are accumulated in a number of specific expense center accounts such as the following:
7-7010		Fiscal Services Administrative Office
		This account is charged with the direct expenses incurred in maintaining the administrative office of the director of fiscal services, including the fees of independent accountants for audit and financial consulting services.
7-7015		General Accounting
7-7020		Budgets and Costs
7-7025		Payroll Accounting
7-7030		Accounts Payable Accounting
7-7035		Plant and Equipment Accounting
7-7040		Inventory Accounting
		These expense centers (7-7015 through 7-7040) perform general accounting, that is, nonpatient billing and accounting activities of the hospital, including preparation of ledgers, budgets, and financial reports; payroll accounting; accounts payable accounting; plant and equipment accounting; inventory accounting; and accounting for tuition, sales to other organizations, and so forth.
		These expense centers should be charged with the direct expenses incurred in fulfilling the general internal accounting requirements of the hospital.
7-7045		Patients' Accounts
		The processing of patient charges, including the processing of charges to patients' accounts, preparing claims, and other

Account Numbers

Expenses Revenues

patient-related billing and accounting activities, is performed by this responsibility center. This expense center should be charged with the direct expenses incurred in patient-related billing and accounting activities.

7-7050 Admitting

The admitting of patients for hospital services includes filling out admission forms, scheduling admission times, accompanying patients to rooms or service areas after admission, and arrangement of admission details. This expense center should be charged with the direct expenses incurred in operating the admitting offices.

7-7055 Cashiering

This department receives and processes payments from or on behalf of patients for hospital and medical services rendered. Additional activities can include, but are not limited to: recording amounts received, examining charges and credit slips to detect errors in posting to patients' accounts, correcting these errors, computing total bills for discharged patients, explaining charges and answering questions concerning accounts, referring patients to the credit department when appropriate, totaling and reconciling cash on a daily basis, preparing deposits, preparing reports of daily transactions, and receiving and storing patients' valuables.

This expense center should be charged with the direct expenses incurred in performing the cashiering function.

7-7060 Credit and Collections

The extension of credit and the collection of accounts receivable are the responsibility of this department. Additional activities include interviewing patients and others concerning the extension of credit, checking references, and using outside collection services.

The provision for bad debts is an expense of this department (the distinction between bad debts and charity service is discussed in the definition of account 5-2101), and the provision for bad debts must be differentiated between inpatient and outpatient services. This can be accomplished by the use of three accounts for the credit and collections department, as follows:

Account Numbers

Expenses Revenues

7-7060 Credit and Collections (excluding bad debts)

7-7061 Provision for Bad Debts—Inpatients

7-7062 Provision for Bad Debts—Outpatients

These expense accounts should be charged with the direct expenses incurred, including bad debts and legal fees related to collection efforts, in extending credit and collecting patients' accounts receivable.

ADMINISTRATIVE SERVICES EXPENSES

7-8000 **Administrative Services**

Administrative services expenses typically are recorded in specific expense center accounts, such as those indicated below:

7-8010 Administrative Offices

This expense center should be charged with the direct expenses of maintaining the administrative offices of the hospital's chief executive officer, including fees for general legal services not related to the collection of accounts or any other specific department or service.

7-8015 Governing Board

Expenses incurred in connection with meetings of the governing board and expenses incurred by the governing board in connection with their hospital-related activities (such as travel expenses) are recorded in this expense center account.

7-8020 Auxiliary Groups

This expense center account is charged with the direct expenses incurred in connection with hospital auxiliary or volunteer groups, including expenses incurred by the coordinator of auxiliary group activities and expenses incurred in connection with special meetings of the auxiliary groups conducted by the hospital.

Account Numbers

Expenses Revenues

7-8025 Chaplaincy Services

This expense center account is charged with the direct expenses of maintaining a chapel for patients and visitors.

7-8030 Public Relations and Development

The public relations and development department furnishes information for public use that aids in promoting and maintaining the hospital's position in the community. It also performs fund raising activities such as special luncheons and other meetings and special mailings.

This expense center account is charged with the direct expenses incurred by the public relations function and with the direct expenses associated with development activities.

7-8035 Purchasing

The purchasing service includes the procuring of supplies, equipment, and services necessary to hospital operations. Additional activities can include, but are not limited to: receipt and processing of requisitions, monitoring perpetual supply items, obtaining quotes from vendors, and monitoring receipt of supplies. This expense center should be charged with the direct expenses incurred in performing the purchasing function.

7-8040 Communications

The communications department operates the communications systems within and outside the hospital, including the telephone system, radio communications systems, public address systems, closed-circuit television, messenger services, and mail processing. This expense center should be charged with the direct expenses incurred in performing the communications function.

7-8045 Information Services

The information services (data processing) department operates the hospital electronic data processing system. This work includes inputing data, storing and safeguarding data, operating data processing equipment, scheduling data processing jobs, distributing output, and identifying and solving hardware and software problems.

Account Numbers

Expenses Revenues

This expense center should be charged with the direct expenses incurred in operating an electronic data processing system. Expenses incurred by the operation of terminals throughout the hospital should be charged to this account. However, outside service bureau costs that are directly identifiable with another expense center's Other Purchased Services natural classification (.60). Outside service bureau costs benefiting more than one expense center should be charged to account 7-8045 and then be allocated in the periodic cost finding.

7-8050 Printing and Duplicating

This department provides printing and duplication of forms, reports, and other printed matter to be used in the hospital. This expense center should be charged with the direct expenses incurred in the operation of a printing and duplicating department.

7-8055 Receiving and Stores

This department receives, stores, and delivers materials, equipment, and supplies to various departments of the hospital. This expense center should be charged with the direct expenses incurred in performing the receiving and stores function.

7-8060 Personnel

The personnel department provides adequate staffing of hospital departments, and promotes employee satisfaction and morale. Activities include recruitment, employee selection, salary and wage administration, fringe benefit program administration, and procurement of temporary workers. This expense center should be charged with the direct expenses incurred in performing the personnel function.

7-8065 Employee Medical Services

The management, administration, and operation of medical services for employees, including scheduling of visits, record keeping in connection with employee visits, and pre-employment and post-illness employee physicals, are included in this expense center. This expense center account should be charged with the direct expenses incurred in operating an employee medical services office or program.

Account Numbers

Expenses Revenues

7-8070 Medical Care Evaluation

The medical care evaluation function includes providing peer review, quality assurance, utilization review, professional standards review, and other medical care evaluation activities. This expense center should be charged with the direct expenses incurred in performing the medical care evaluation activities.

RESEARCH AND EDUCATION EXPENSES

6.9 The accounts used to record the expenses associated with hospital research projects and educational programs are described in Figure 6-5.

Figure 6-5
Research and Education Expenses

Account Numbers		
Expenses	Revenues	
		RESEARCH EXPENSES
8-1000		**Research**
		This series of accounts is used to record the direct expenses incurred by the hospital in its medical research activities. The expense centers carry on research projects funded by outside donations or grants and/or the hospital. Additional activities include maintenance of the animal house and the administration of specific research projects. These expense centers should be charged with the direct expenses incurred in performing research in the hospital. Separate expense center accounts must be maintained for each research activity for which a separate accounting is required either by a grant agreement or contract or because of restrictions imposed by donors or grantors.
8-1010		Administrative Office
		The overall administration and management of research projects carried on by the hospital are performed by the research administrative office. Administrative expenses related to specific research projects or groups of projects should be recorded in the expense center related to that project or group of projects.
8-1200		Hospital Research Projects
8-1300		Joint Research Projects
8-1400		Medical School Research Projects
		EDUCATION EXPENSES
8-4000		**Education**
		This series of accounts is used to record the direct expenses of educational programs carried on by the hospital.

Account Numbers

Expenses Revenues

8-4010 Administrative Office

The overall administration and management of all educational programs and activities carried on by the hospital are performed by the education administrative office.

8-4100 **Nursing and Allied Health Education**

This series of accounts is charged with the direct expenses related to nonphysician educational programs and activities such as a school of nursing or a school of laboratory technology.

8-4110 Administrative Office

This expense center account should be charged with the direct expenses incurred in maintaining a nursing and allied health education administrative office.

8-4115 Registered Nurse Program

The school of nursing is an approved, licensed school for the education of registered nurses. Additional activities can include, but are not limited to: selecting qualified nursing students; providing education in theory and practice conforming to approved standards; maintaining student personnel records; counseling students regarding professional, personal, and educational problems; selecting faculty personnel; assigning and supervising students who are involved in providing nursing care to selected patients; and administering aptitude and other tests for counseling and selection purposes. This expense center account should be charged for the direct expenses incurred in operating a school of nursing for registered nurses.

8-4120 Licensed Practical Nurse Program

The licensed vocational nurse program is an approved and licensed school for educating licensed practical nurses. Additional activities can include, but are not limited to: selecting qualified nursing students; providing education in theory and practice conforming to approved standards; maintaining student personnel records; counseling students regarding professional, personal, and educational problems; assigning and supervising students who are involved in providing nursing care to selected patients; and administering aptitude and other

Account Numbers

Expenses Revenues

tests for counseling and selection purposes. This expense center should be charged with the direct expenses incurred in operating a licensed vocational nurse program.

8-4125 Allied Health Education

Allied health education includes training programs such as cytotechnologist, cardiovascular perfusionist, clinical pastoral counselor, dietetic intern, health services administrator, histologic technician or technologist, medical laboratory technician, medical record technician, nuclear medicine technologist, occupational therapist, pharmacy resident, physical therapist, radiation therapy technologist, and radiographer. Separate accounts may be maintained for each training program.

8-4200 **Graduate Medical Education**

This expense center account is charged with the direct expenses associated with members of the medical staff who are not assigned to specific professional service departments. More specific accounts, as indicated below, can be used to differentiate among the expenses of the voluntary staff, the paid staff, and the medical graduate education staff and student body.

8-4210 Voluntary Medical Staff

This expense center account is charged with the direct expenses associated with the voluntary staff, including expenses for staff meetings and other related activities.

8-4215 Paid Medical Staff

This expense center account is charged with the direct expenses associated with the paid medical staff for the provision of physician services to patients and for supervision thereof. Included are salaries of the chief of medical staff and other chiefs of services, and salaries and other expenses associated with the house medical staff.

8-4220 Interns

Account Numbers

Expenses Revenues

8-4225 Residents

These expense center accounts are charged with the direct expenses of a formally organized medical graduate education program that provides medical graduate clinical education to interns and residents. Additional activities include, but are not limited to: selecting qualified students; providing education in theory and practice conforming to approved standards; maintaining student personnel records; counseling students regarding professional, personal, and educational problems; and assigning and supervising students.

UNASSIGNED EXPENSES

6.10 In addition to the expenses that can be directly identified with and charged to a particular responsibility center, other types of expenses are incurred that are related to two or more responsibility centers. It may not always be convenient, in the regular routine of accounting, to charge these other expenses to the several centers to which they relate. Also, a particular expense (depreciation of the hospital building, for example) may not be subject to control by a single responsibility center manager. As a result, these types of expenses generally are not charged directly to responsibility centers in the routine accounting process, but are instead accumulated in a series of *unassigned expense* accounts. When a cost finding is performed, the unassigned expenses are allocated to the various responsibility centers. These unassigned expenses are described in Figure 6-6.

Figure 6-6
Unassigned Expenses

Account Numbers		
Expenses	Revenues	
8-6100		**Depreciation**
		Depreciation is a system of accounting that aims to distribute the cost or other basic value of tangible capital assets, less salvage (if any), over the estimated useful life of the unit (which may be a group of assets) in a systematic and rational manner.
		The following specific accounts are used to record depreciation expenses by major classes of depreciable assets. Subsidiary plant asset records should be maintained to facilitate the allocation of depreciation expenses equitably to the appropriate responsibility centers in the cost-finding process.
8-6182		Land Improvements
8-6183		Buildings
8-6184		Leasehold Improvements
8-6185		Fixed Equipment
8-6186		Major Movable Equipment
8-6200		**Rent**
		This account is used to record rent expenses (including expenses arising from operating leases) that is not directly and easily assignable to responsibility centers in the regular accounting routine.
8-6300		**Insurance**
		This account is charged with all insurance expenses (except employee benefit insurance, which is charged to account 8-7100) that is not directly and easily chargeable to responsibility centers in the regular accounting routine. General legal malpractice insurance should be charged to this account.
8-6400		**Interest**

Account Numbers		
Expenses	Revenues	
8-6410		Working Capital Interest
		This account is charged with interest incurred on borrowings to finance temporary working capital needs.
8-6415		Other Interest
		This account is charged with interest incurred on borrowings for other than working capital purposes. Interest incurred on mortgages and loans made for the acquisition of equipment should be included in this account. Interest expenses arising from capital leases also should be charged to this account.
8-7100		**Employee Benefits**
		This account is charged for the employer's share of employee benefit costs. Separate accounts, such as indicated below, should be maintained for each type of employee benefit:
8-7110		Social Security Taxes
8-7115		Federal and State Unemployment Taxes
8-7120		Group Health and Life Insurance
8-7125		Retirement Plan Expense
8-7130		Workmen's Compensation Insurance
8-7135		Group Disability Insurance
8-7200		**Housing**
8-7210		Student Housing
		The student housing service maintains residences for students participating in educational programs carried on by the hospital. This account should be charged for the direct costs incurred in providing housing for those students.
8-7215		Employee Housing
		The employee housing service maintains residences for employees. This account should be charged with the direct expenses incurred in providing housing to those employees.

Account Numbers

Expenses Revenues

8-7220 Physicians' Offices

This account should be charged with the direct expenses incurred in the provision of rental space to physicians and other professional persons, and in other rental activities such as the rental of movable equipment.

8-7300 **Medical Photography and Illustration**

This account should be charged with the direct expenses incurred by an organized department of medical photography and illustration.

8-7400 **Medical Malpractice Expense**

8-8000 **Taxes**

This series of accounts is used to record all types of taxes paid by the hospital, including income taxes, property taxes, and payments in lieu of taxes.

8-8100 Income Tax Expense

Separate accounts, as indicated below, should be used to obtain the necessary classification of income taxes:

8-8110 Federal Income Tax Expense Currently Payable

8-8115 Provision for Deferred Federal Income Tax

8-8120 State Income Tax Expense Currently Payable

8-8125 Provision for Deferred State Income Tax

8-8200 Property Tax Expense

This account is used to record property taxes assessed by governmental units.

8-9100 Payments in Lieu of Taxes

The hospital may be required to make payments in lieu of taxes to governmental units. Accounting and financial reporting guidelines for such payments are provided in the exposure draft of a proposed P&P Board Statement issued April 1, 1993. In this statement, these payments are grouped into three broad types: payments for governmental services, payments

Account Numbers

Expenses Revenues

into charity pools, and payments for general governmental support. Depending upon the circumstances, certain amounts of these payments should be regarded as payments for general governmental support and should be charged to this expense account.

NONOPERATING GAINS AND LOSSES

6.11 As discussed in Chapter 2 (starting at paragraph 23), revenues and expenses arise only from hospital activities that constitute the hospital's ongoing major or central operations. All revenues are operating revenues; all expenses are operating expenses. Gains and losses, however, may be classified and reported as either operating or nonoperating, depending upon the individual hospital's definition of its ongoing major or central operations and how the gains or losses relate to that definition.

6.12 As a result, particular gains or losses may properly be recorded by some hospitals as revenues (see Chapter 6, paragraph 7 and Figure 6-3) while other hospitals may properly record the same types of gains or losses as nonoperating gains or losses. Figure 6-7 provides a listing of accounts for nonoperating gains and losses, assuming a definition of "ongoing major or central operations" that may be appropriate for some hospitals. Other hospitals would need to adjust the chart of accounts to include certain of these gains and losses in revenues (the 5-0000 series of accounts). Similarly, some hospitals would need to adjust the illustrative chart of accounts to transfer certain revenue accounts to the nonoperating gains classification.

Figure 6-7
Nonoperating Gains and Losses

Account Numbers

Expenses Revenues

9-1000 **Unrestricted Gifts and Bequests**

This account is used to record the receipt of cash and other resources from donors who place no restrictions on the use of the resources.

9-2000 **Income and Gains (Losses) on Investments**

9-2100 Investments of Unrestricted Resources

This account is used to record interest income, dividend income, and gains (losses) on sales of investments of unrestricted resources. Subaccounts should be established to distinguish between gains and losses.

9-2200 Investments of Restricted Resources

This account is used to record interest income, dividend income, and gains (losses) on sales of investments of restricted resources, but only if the income or gains are unrestricted by donors. Subaccounts should be established to identify the particular group of restricted resources (fund) and to distinguish between gains and losses.

9-2300 Investments Whose Use Is Limited

This account is used to record interest income, dividend income, and gains (losses) on sales of investments of resources whose use is limited, but only if the use of the income or gains is not also limited by contract or other agreement.

9-3000 **Gains (Losses) on Disposal of Plant Assets**

This account is used to record gains (losses) on sales of plant assets, including land, buildings, and equipment.

OTHER ACCOUNTS

6.13 There may be an occasional need to include certain special items in the hospital statement of income and other changes in unrestricted equity. The 9-9000 series of accounts, indicated in Figure 6-8, is available to record those items.

Figure 6-8
Other Accounts

Account Numbers

Expenses Revenues

9-9100 **Gain (Loss) on Disposal of a Business Segment**

This account is used to record the gain (loss) on the disposal of a segment of the hospital business (such as a separate long-term care facility owned by the hospital) in accordance with the requirements of APB Opinion No. 30.[2]

9-9200 **Extraordinary Gains (Losses)**

This account is used to record extraordinary gains (losses) in accordance with the requirements of APB Opinion No. 30.[3] An extraordinary gain (loss) may arise, for example, from the early extinguishment of debt (bonds payable) or as a result of a major casualty such as an earthquake.

9-9300 **Cumulative Effect on Prior Years of Change in an Accounting Principle**

This account is used to record the cumulative effect on the net income of prior periods of a change from one generally accepted accounting principle to another accounting principle as a gain (loss) in the income statement of the year of change as required by APB Opinion No. 20.[4]

2 APB Opinion No. 30, *Reporting the Results of Operations* (AICPA: New York, 1973).

3 Ibid.

4 APB Opinion No. 20, *Accounting Changes* (AICPA: New York, 1971). A change from one method of depreciation to another, for example, may require the use of this account.

7

Illustrative Financial Statements

7.1 Financial statements are the end products of the accounting process. They provide quantitative information about an entity's financial position, operating results, and cash flows. This information is necessary for the effective management of an entity, and it is also essential to external users such as investors, donors, and creditors.

7.2 This chapter presents a complete set of financial statements for external general-purpose reporting by a hospital. The statements reflect the applications of the accounting and reporting principles discussed in this book. The statements are illustrative only. Other formats, other types of disclosure, and other levels of detail may be employed. Other classifications also may be appropriate, depending on how an individual hospital defines its ongoing major or central activities in its mission statement. For example, unrestricted contributions from donors may be reported as revenues by one hospital but as nonoperating (peripheral or incidental) gains by another hospital.

7.3 The illustrative statements (and accompanying notes) are similar to those included in Appendix A of the AICPA audit and accounting guide.[1] In addition, the illustrative statements and notes reflect the requirements of FASB Statement of Financial Accounting Standards No. 117.[2] Neither the illustrations in this chapter nor those in the AICPA guide and FASB statement are intended to prescribe a single acceptable model for the presentation of financial information. Differences between the financial statement illustrations in this book and those in the AICPA and FASB

1 *Audits of Providers of Health Care Services* (New York: AICPA, 1990), appendix A, pp. 145-206.

2 Statement of Financial Accounting Standards No. 117, *Financial Statements of Not-for-Profit Organizations* (Norwalk, Connecticut: FASB, 1993).

documents do not evidence any disagreement concerning financial statement format or content but do demonstrate generally acceptable display alternatives. However, a basic consistency between governmental and nongovernmental entities in accounting principles and reporting practices is essential.

BALANCE SHEETS

7.4 Balance sheets (sometimes called statements of financial position) present the financial position of a hospital in terms of its assets, liabilities, and equity (net assets) at a given point in time. The definitions of these elements of the balance sheet appear in paragraphs 19 through 22 of Chapter 2.

7.5 Comparative balance sheets for Hypothetical Hospital are provided in Figure 7-1. These balance sheets are presented in an aggregated format. The AICPA and the FASB have indicated that reporting of assets and liabilities classified by funds is not a necessary part of general-purpose external financial reporting. In addition, the HFMA Principles and Practices Board has recommended that the general-purpose financial statements of hospitals present all assets, liabilities, and equity in a single aggregated balance sheet without differentiation by fund.[3]

7.6 When a fund accounting system is used and the aggregated balance sheet format is adopted, the assets of the donor-restricted funds (excluding interfund receivables) are merged with the assets of the unrestricted (general) fund. The liabilities of the donor-restricted funds (excluding interfund liabilities) are combined with the liabilities of the unrestricted fund. Corresponding amounts of cash balances are adjusted as if the interfund receivables and liabilities had been settled.

7.7 In Figure 7-1, the hospital's equity is presented in three parts as discussed at paragraphs 2.22 and 5.37: (1) unrestricted equity, (2) temporarily donor-restricted equity, and (3) permanently donor-restricted equity. When a fund accounting system is used, the temporarily donor-restricted equity is the sum of the equity (fund balances) of the specific purpose, plant replacement and expansion, and term endowment funds; the permanently donor-restricted equity is the equity (fund balances) of the permanent endowment funds.

3 Principles and Practices Board Statement No. 8, *The Use of Fund Accounting and the Need for Single Fund Reporting by Institutional Healthcare Providers* (Westchester, Illlinois: HFMA, 1984).

Figure 7-1
HYPOTHETICAL HOSPITAL
Balance Sheets
December 31, 1994 and 1993
(Dollar Amounts in Thousands)

	12/31/94	12/31/93
ASSETS		
Current assets:		
Cash and cash equivalents	$ 4,152	$ 3,202
Short-term investments, at cost which approximates market	814	677
Assets whose use is limited, and required for current liabilities (notes 5 and 7)	1,219	1,174
Patient accounts receivable, net	14,920	14,544
Inventories	1,297	1,063
Other current assets	617	641
Total current assets	23,019	21,301
Investment in Affiliated Entity (note 4)	855	450
Assets whose use is limited or donor-restricted, net of amount required for current liabilities (notes 5, 7, 9)	37,922	34,406
Property, plant, and equipment, net (notes 6, 7)	52,935	50,848
Other assets	946	1,008
Total assets	$115,677	$108,013

LIABILITIES AND EQUITY

Current liabilities:		
Current portion of long-term debt (note 7) and estimated malpractice costs (note 8)	$ 1,490	$ 1,536
Accounts payable	2,564	2,643
Accrued expenses payable	3,509	3,317
Estimated third-party payor settlements—Medicaid (note 3)	2,086	1,884
Other current liabilities	1,472	1,962
Total current liabilities	11,121	11,334
Long-term debt, net of current portion (notes 7, 8)	24,181	25,296
Estimated malpractice costs, net of current portion (note 8)	2,903	2,264
Deferred third-party revenues	814	987
Commitments and contingent liabilities (notes 3, 6, 8, 12, 13)		
Total liabilities	39,019	39,881
Equity:		
Unrestricted	67,515	61,970
Temporarily donor-restricted	5,802	4,115
Permanently donor-restricted	3,341	2,047
Total equity	76,658	68,132
Total liabilities and equity	$115,677	$108,013

The accompanying notes are an integral part of these financial statements. (Illustrative notes appear in Figure 7-7.)

STATEMENTS OF INCOME AND OTHER CHANGES IN UNRESTRICTED EQUITY

7.8 Statements of income and other changes in unrestricted equity present the changes in unrestricted equity in terms of revenues, assets released from restrictions, expenses, gains, and losses for a specified period of time. The elements of this financial statement are defined in Chapter 2, paragraphs 23 through 27.

7.9 Figure 7-2 provides illustrative statements of income and other changes in unrestricted equity for Hypothetical Hospital. The format employed here is only one of several alternatives presented in FASB Statement No. 117. It should be noted that Statement No. 117 does not permit the presentation of the traditional income statement in external general-purpose financial reporting by not-for-profit organizations. The statement shown in Figure 7-2 amounts to a combined income statement and statement of changes in unrestricted equity (net assets), but without any line item for *net income*. For internal managerial reporting and certain other purposes, the development and use of traditional income statements is recommended.

Figure 7-2
HYPOTHETICAL HOSPITAL
Statement of Income and Other Changes in Unrestricted Equity
Years Ended December 31, 1994 and 1993
(Dollar Amounts in Thousands)

	1994	1993
Revenues:		
Patient service revenues (note 3)	$ 93,850	$ 88,162
Other revenues	9,033	7,844
Total revenues	102,883	96,006
Net assets released from restrictions	354	409
Total revenues and other support	103,237	96,415
Expenses (notes 7, 8, 12, and 14):		
Salaries and wages	48,492	47,129
Employee benefits	9,772	8,909
Professional fees	4,825	4,208
Supplies and materials	16,284	15,773
Purchased services	10,878	9,766
Medical malpractice costs	915	568
Depreciation	4,357	4,092
Interest	1,859	1,977
Provision for bad debts	1,015	1,206
Other	323	419
Total expenses	98,720	94,047

Income from operations	4,517	1,618
Gains (losses):		
Investment gains	1,070	819
Loss on investment in Affiliated Entity	(42)	(26)
Net gains	1,028	793
Increase in unrestricted equity	5,545	2,411
Unrestricted equity at beginning of year	61,970	59,559
Unrestricted equity at end of year	$ 67,515	$ 61,970

The accompanying notes are an integral part of these financial statements. (Illustrative notes appear in Figure 7-7.)

Revenues

7.10 Patient service revenues are measured and reported in the amounts expected to be collected from patients and their third-party sponsors for healthcare services provided by the hospital, i.e., the amounts patients and third-parties have an obligation to pay. In other words, revenues represent actual or expected cash inflows.

7.11 This means that reported revenues should exclude charges related to contractual adjustments and charity care. The amounts of contractual adjustments and charity care do not appear in the body of the statement but are disclosed in notes accompanying the financial statements. Such a note is illustrated in Figure 7-7 (Note 2).

7.12 In addition to patient service revenues, the statement reports "other revenues." Depending upon the hospital's definition of its ongoing major or central activities (see paragraphs 23 and 26 of Chapter 2), "other revenues" could include such items as:

- Revenues arising from unrestricted gifts and from unrestricted income from investments of restricted resources.

- Revenues from sources such as tuition from educational programs, cafeteria, sales, parking fees, television rentals, and vending machine commissions. (A more complete listing appears in Chapter 4.)

- Investment income on malpractice or other trust funds.

A hospital that defines its ongoing major or central activities in a different way might appropriately report certain of these items as nonoperating gains.

Assets Released from Restrictions

7.13 Receipts of contributions that are donor-restricted for a specific purpose (such as research, education, charity care, plant asset acquisitions, and term endowments) are reported in the statement of changes in equity (see Figure 7-3) in the period received as an increase in temporarily donor-restricted equity. When the donor restrictions are fulfilled, these amounts are "assets released from restrictions" (sometimes referred to as "other support"), and are reclassified as additions to unrestricted equity in the statement of income and other changes in unrestricted equity as shown in Figure 7-2. In the same period, these amounts also are reported as deductions from temporarily donor-restricted equity in the statement of changes in equity as shown in Figure 7-3.

7.14 Contributions that are donor-restricted to permanent endowments are reported in the statement of changes in equity in the period received as an increase in permanently donor-restricted equity. Except in extremely rare circumstances, these amounts are not reclassified at a later date as additions to unrestricted equity.

Expenses

7.15 The expenses in Figure 7-2 are presented in a natural (object of expenditure) classification rather than in a functional classification. A functional classification of expenses, however, should be disclosed in the notes accompanying the financial statements (see note 14 in Figure 7-7). All expenses are reductions of unrestricted equity.

Nonoperating Gains and Losses

7.16 The individually significant nonoperating gains and losses are separately listed as illustrated in Figure 7-2. Depending on the hospital's definition of its ongoing major and central activities, this classification also may include items such as:

- Tax levies and other subsidies from governmental or community agencies received for the general support of the hospital;
- Gains and losses on sales of plant assets and investments of unrestricted assets; and
- Net rentals of facilities that are not used in hospital operating activities.

7.17 In Figures 7-2 and 7-3, it is assumed that income and gains (losses) arising from investments of temporarily donor-restricted resources also are donor-restricted. In addition, it is assumed that income arising from investments of permanently donor-restricted resources is not donor-restricted, but that gains (losses) arising from investments of those resources are donor-restricted.

STATEMENTS OF CHANGES IN EQUITY

7.18 A statement of changes in equity (net assets) reports the changes (increases and decreases) that have occurred during a specified period of time in the hospital's unrestricted equity, temporarily donor-restricted equity, and permanently donor-restricted equity. Figure 7-3 provides an illustration of statements of changes in equity (layered or "pancake" format) for Hypothetical Hospital. One alternative to the layered format is the columnar format shown in Figure 7-4 (comparative data for 1993 are not included for the sake of simplicity).

Figure 7-3
HYPOTHETICAL HOSPITAL
Statements of Changes in Equity
Years Ended December 31, 1994 and 1993
(Dollar Amounts in Thousands)

	1994	1993
Unrestricted equity:		
Total revenues	$ 102,883	$ 96,006
Assets released from restrictions	354	409
Total expenses	(98,720)	(94,797)
Gains (net of losses)	1,028	793
Increase in unrestricted equity	5,545	2,411
Temporarily donor-restricted equity:		
Contributions	1,786	647
Investment income	255	202
Net assets released from restrictions	(354)	(409)
Increase in temporarily donor-restricted equity	1,687	440
Permanently donor-restricted equity:		
Contributions	994	750
Net unrealized and realized investment gains	300	
Net unrealized and realized investment losses		(266)
Increase in permanently donor-restricted equity	1,294	484
Total increase in equity	8,526	3,335
Total equity at beginning of year	68,132	64,797
Equity at end of year	$ 76,658	$ 68,132

The accompanying notes are an integral part of these financial statements. (Illustrative notes appear in Figure 7-7.)

Figure 7-4
HYPOTHETICAL HOSPITAL
Statement of Changes in Equity
Year Ended December 31, 1994
(Dollar Amounts in Thousands)

	Un-restricted	Temporarily Donor-Restricted	Permanently Donor-Restricted	Total
Revenues, gains, and other support:				
Unrestricted revenues	$102,883			$102,883
Unrestricted gains, net	1,070			1,070
Restricted revenues, gains, and other support:				
Contributions		$ 1,786	$ 994	2,780
Investment income		255		255
Net unrealized and realized gains on investments			300	300
Assets released from restrictions	354	(354)		
Total revenues, gains, and other support	104,307	1,687	1,294	107,288
Expenses and losses:				
Expenses	98,720			98,720
Loss on investment in Affiliated Entity	42			42
Total expenses and losses	98,762			98,762

	Un-restricted	Temporarily Donor-Restricted	Permanently Donor-Restricted	Total
Increase in equity	5,545	1,687	1,294	8,526
Equity at beginning of year	61,970	4,115	2,047	68,132
Equity at end of year	$67,515	$ 5,802	$ 3,341	$76,658

(Accompanying notes are not provided for this statement.)

STATEMENTS OF CASH FLOWS

7.19 Figures 7-5 and 7-6 present Hypothetical Hospital's statements of cash flows. The primary purpose of these statements is to provide a complete summary of all of the inflows and outflows of the hospital's cash and cash equivalents (both unrestricted and restricted) during a specified period of time. The information in statements of cash flows, if used with related disclosures and information in the other financial statements, should assist investors, creditors, and others in assessing:

- The hospital's ability to generate positive future net cash flows;
- The hospital's ability to meet its obligations;
- The hospital's need for external financing;
- The reasons for differences between the change in net assets and associated cash receipts and cash payments; and
- The effects on the hospital's financial position of its operating, investing, and financing activities.

For this purpose, the term *cash* includes cash equivalents, which consist of short-term, highly liquid investments that are readily convertible into known amounts of cash and have an original maturity of three months or less.[4]

Classification of Cash Flows

7.20 In the statement of cash flows, cash receipts and cash payments are classified into three categories:

- *Cash Flows from Operating Activities.* Operating activities include the transactions that result in revenues, expenses, and gains and losses.
- *Cash Flows from Investing Activities.* Investing activities include making and collecting loans; acquiring and disposing of investments in securities; and acquiring and disposing of property, plant, and equipment.
- *Cash Flows from Financing Activities.* Financing activities include borrowings, repayment of borrowings, and donor-restricted contributions.

Certain cash flows relating to investing and financing activities are included in the operating activities classification. For example, a borrowing of money is a financing activity, but a payment of interest to the lender is an operating activity. Similarly,

4 Statement of Financial Accounting Standards No. 95, *Statement of Cash Flows* (Stamford, Connecticut: FASB, 1987). Also see FASB Statement No. 117, pp.64-67.

an investment in securities is an investing activity, but a receipt of interest or dividend income is reported as a cash inflow from operating activities.

7.21 The Governmental Accounting Standards Board has prescribed a statement of cash flows that has some similarities to the statement required by the FASB, but also has significant differences.[5] One major difference is that the GASB provides for four categories of cash flows: (1) operating activities, (2) noncapital financing activities, (3) capital and related financing activities, and (4) investing activities. Also, GASB defines the cash flow categories differently from the FASB even though using some of the same category names. The GASB statement of cash flows, however, is not illustrated in this book.

Reporting Cash Flows from Operating Activities

7.22 There are two methods of reporting cash flows from operating activities: the *indirect method* and the *direct method*. The indirect method is illustrated in Figure 7-5; the direct method is illustrated in Figure 7-6.

7.23 *Indirect Method*. The indirect method starts with the reported change in equity and converts it into net cash flow from operating activities by adjusting the change in equity for items that were included in the determination of the change in equity but did not affect cash (and cash equivalents).

7.24 *Direct Method*. Under the direct method, the cash flows from operating activities are presented in what amounts to a cash-basis income statement. A supporting schedule is required to reconcile the net cash flow from operating activities with the reported change in equity.

Reporting Significant Noncash Transactions

7.25 The body of the statement of cash flows includes only those transactions and events that resulted in cash flows. However, there generally are significant transactions and events that do not involve cash but are investing or financing activities, e.g., exchanges of nonmonetary assets and acquisition of assets by assuming liabilities (including capital lease obligations). Transactions such as these should be disclosed either by a note to the statement of cash flows or in a schedule at the bottom of the statement.

5 *Reporting Cash Flows of Proprietary and Nonexpendable Trust Funds and Governmental Entities That Use Proprietary Accounting* (Norwalk, Connecticut: GASB, 1989).

Figure 7-5
HYPOTHETICAL HOSPITAL
Statements of Cash Flows
(Indirect Method)
Years Ended December 31, 1994 and 1993

	1994	1993
Cash flows from operating activities:		
Increase in equity	$ 8,526	$ 3,335
Adjustments to reconcile increase in net assets to net cash provided by operating activities:		
Depreciation and amortization	4,357	4,092
Provision for uncollectible patient accounts	1,015	1,206
Loss on investment in Affiliated Entity	42	26
Net realized and unrealized gains on investments	(1,370)	(553)
Increase (decrease) in amounts due to third-party payors	29	179
Increase (decrease) in liability for estimated malpractice costs	639	(235)
Increase in patient accounts receivable	(1,391)	(274)
Increase in supplies and other assets	(148)	(110)
Increase (decrease) in accounts payable, accrued expenses, and other liabilities	(305)	251
Increase in interest earned but not received on assets whose use is limited	(23)	(18)
Net cash provided by operating activities	11,371	7,899

Cash flows from investing activities:		
Purchase of property and equipment	(6,444)	(5,081)
Sales of investments		249
Purchases of investments	(137)	
Investment in Affiliated Entity	(447)	(476)
Cash invested in assets whose use is limited	(2,168)	(873)
Net cash used in investing activities	(9,196)	(6,181)
Cash flows from financing activities:		
Repayment of long-term debt	(1,225)	(1,090)
Net cash used in financing activities	(1,225)	(1,090)
Net increase (decrease) in cash and cash equivalents	950	628
Cash and cash equivalents, beginning of year	3,202	2,574
Cash and cash equivalents, end of year	$ 4,152	$ 3,202

The accompanying notes are an integral part of these financial statements. (Illustrative notes appear in Figure 7-7.)

Figure 7-6
HYPOTHETICAL HOSPITAL
Statements of Cash Flows
(Direct Method)
Years Ended December 31, 1994 and 1993

	1994	1993
Cash flows from operating activities:		
Cash received from patients and third-party payors	$ 94,226	$ 88,989
Cash paid to employees and suppliers	(92,278)	(88,207)
Cash received from contributors and grantors	4,392	1,535
Other receipts from operations	4,219	5,043
Interest and dividends received	2,592	2,395
Interest paid (net of amount capitalized)	(1,780)	(1,856)
Net cash provided by operating activities	11,371	7,899
Cash flows from investing activities:		
Purchases of property and equipment	(6,444)	(5,081)
Sales of investments		249
Purchases of investments	(137)	
Investment in Affiliated Entity	(447)	(476)
Cash invested in assets whose use is limited	(2,168)	(873)
Net cash used in investing activities	(9,196)	(6,181)
Cash flows from financing activities:		
Repayment of long-term debt	(1,225)	(1,090)

Net cash used in financing activities	(1,225)	(1,090)
Net increase in cash and cash equivalents	950	628
Cash and cash equivalents, beginning of year	3,202	2,574
Cash and cash equivalents, end of year	**$ 4,152**	**$ 3,202**

Reconciliation of increase in equity to net cash provided by operating activities:	1994	1993
Increase in equity	$ 8,526	$ 3,335
Adjustments to reconcile increase in net assets to net cash provided by operating activities:		
Depreciation and amortization	4,357	4,092
Provision for uncollectible patient accounts	1,015	1,206
Loss on investment in Affiliated Entity	42	26
Net realized and unrealized gains on investments	(1,370)	(553)
Increase (decrease) in amounts due to third-party payors	29	179
Increase (decrease) in liability for estimated malpractice costs	639	(235)
Increase in patient accounts receivable	(1,391)	(274)
Increase in supplies and current assets	(148)	(110)
Increase (decrease) in accounts payable, accrued expenses payable, and other liabilities	(305)	251
Increase in interest earned but not received on assets whose use is limited	(23)	(18)
Net cash provided by operating activities	**$ 11,371**	**$ 7,899**

(Accompanying notes are not illustrated for this financial statement.)

NOTES ACCOMPANYING THE FINANCIAL STATEMENTS

7.26 Notes are an integral part of the financial statements of the hospital, and this should be stated at the foot of each financial statement included in the hospital's annual report. Notes are used to amplify or explain the information presented in the financial statements. Figure 7-7 presents an illustrative (but not comprehensive) set of notes to accompany the aggregated financial statements of Hypothetical Hospital presented earlier in Figures 7-1, 7-2, 7-3, and 7-5. These notes are adapted (with permission) from those appearing in the AICPA's health care audit guide.[6]

6 *Audits of Providers of Health Care Services* (New York: AICPA, 1990), pp. 157-166.

Figure 7-7
HYPOTHETICAL HOSPITAL
Notes to Accompany Financial Statements
Years Ended December 31, 1994 and 1993

1. Summary of Significant Accounting Policies.

Organization. Hypothetical Hospital (Hospital) is a not-for-profit hospital. The Hospital, incorporated in the State of Indiana, provides acute health care services. Effective June 30, 1993, under a reorganization plan, Goodcare Health System was formed as the parent holding company of the Hospital. Goodcare Health System has the authority to appoint Hospital trustees, approve major Hospital expenditures, and approve long-term borrowings by the Hospital.

Charity Care. The Hospital provides care to patients who meet certain criteria under its charity care policy without charge or at amounts less than its established rates. Amounts that qualify as charity care are not reported as receivables or revenues.

Income Taxes. The Hospital is a not-for-profit corporation as described in Section 501(c)(3) of the Internal Revenue Code and is exempt from federal income taxes on related income pursuant to Section 501(a) of the Code.

Patient Service Revenues. Patient service revenues are reported at the estimated realizable amounts from patients, third-party payors, and others for services rendered, including estimated retroactive adjustments under agreements with third-party payors. Retroactive adjustments are accrued on an estimated basis in the period the related services are rendered and adjusted in future periods as final settlements are determined.

Investments and Investment Income. Donated investments received are reported at fair value at the date of receipt, which is thereafter treated as cost. Marketable equity securities included in investment portfolios are carried at market value at the balance sheet date. The Hospital's investment in Affiliated Entity is reported on the equity method of accounting that approximates the Hospital's equity in the underlying net book value of Affiliated Entity. Substantially all marketable debt securities are carried at amortized cost in that the Hospital has both the intent and the ability to hold those securities to maturity.

Investment income on proceeds of borrowings that are held by a trustee, to the extent not capitalized, and investment income on assets deposited in a malpractice trust are reported as other revenues. Investment income from all other unrestricted investments are reported as nonoperating gains. Investment income and gains (losses) on investments of donor-restricted resources, including endowments, are reported as nonoperating gains or are added to (deducted from) donor-restricted equity in conformity with each donor's stipulations.

Pledges. Donor unconditional commitments to contribute amounts in future years (pledges), less an allowance for uncollectible amounts, are recorded as receivables in the year made. Pledges whose eventual collection is not reasonably assured are not recorded. Unrestricted pledges are reported as operating gains; restricted pledges are reported as assets and as additions to restricted equity.

Statement of Income and Other Changes in Unrestricted Equity. For purposes of display, transactions deemed by Hospital management to be ongoing major or central to the provision of health care services are reported as revenues and expenses. Peripheral or incidental amounts are reported as gains and losses.

Borrowing Costs. Interest incurred on borrowed funds during the period of construction of plant assets is capitalized as a component of the cost of those plant assets. Deferred financing costs are amortized over the period the related obligation is outstanding using the interest method. Amortization of deferred financing costs is capitalized during the period of construction of plant assets.

Donated Resources. Donor-restricted resources are those whose use is restricted by donors. Unrestricted resources are those on which donors have placed no restriction or that arise as a result of the operations of the Hospital for its stated purposes. Receipts of restricted resources are reported as increases in donor-restricted equity in the statement of changes in equity. When the donor restrictions are fulfilled, the amount of resources so released from restrictions is reported as an increase in unrestricted equity in the statement of income and other changes in unrestricted equity. Receipts of unrestricted resources are reported as other revenues.

Resources restricted by donors to permanent endowment are reported as increases in permanently donor-restricted equity.

Assets Whose Use Is Limited. Assets whose use is limited include assets set aside by the Hospital's Board of Trustees for future capital improvements, over which the Board retains control and may at its discretion use for any purpose; assets set aside in accordance with agreements with third-party payors; and assets held by trustees under bond indenture agreements and self-insurance trust arrangements.

Property, Plant, and Equipment. Property, plant, and equipment acquisitions are recorded at cost. Property, plant, and equipment donated for hospital operations are recorded as additions to restricted equity at fair value at the date of receipt, and as additions to unrestricted equity the assets are placed in service.

Depreciation is computed by the straight-line method over the estimated useful life of each class of depreciable assets. Equipment acquired under capital leases is depreciated by the straight-line method over the estimated useful life of the equipment or the lease term, whichever is the shorter period.

Cash and Cash Equivalents. Cash equivalents include investments in highly liquid debt instruments with an original maturity of three months or less.

Estimated Malpractice Costs. The provision for estimated self-insured medical malpractice claims includes estimates of the ultimate costs for both reported claims and claims incurred but not reported.

2. **Charity Care.**

The Hospital maintains records to identify and monitor the level of charity care it provides. These records include the amount of charges foregone for services and supplies furnished under its charity care policy, the estimated cost of those services and supplies, and equivalent service statistics. The following information indicates the level of charity care provided during 1994 and 1993 (dollar amounts are in thousands):

	1994	1993
Charges foregone, based on established rates	$5,643	$5,128
Estimated expenses incurred to provide charity care	$5,216	$4,709
Equivalent percentage of charity services to all services provided	5.9%	5.8%

3. Patient Service Revenues.

The Hospital has agreements with third-party payors that provide for payments to the Hospital at amounts different from its established rates. A summary of the payment arrangements with major third-party payors is provided below:

Medicare. Inpatient acute care services rendered to Medicare program beneficiaries under a local plan are paid at prospectively determined rates per discharge.

These rates vary according to a patient classification system that is based on clinical, diagnostic, and other factors. Inpatient nonacute services, certain outpatient services, and medical education costs related to Medicare beneficiaries are paid based on actual costs incurred. A tentative payment is received during the year for items paid on a cost basis with final settlement determined after submission of annual cost reports by the Hospital and audits thereof by the Medicare fiscal intermediary. The Hospital's classification of patients under the Medicare program and the appropriateness of their admission are subject to an independent review by a peer review organization under contract with the Hospital. The Hospital's Medicare cost reports have been audited by the Medicare fiscal intermediary through December 31, 1991.

Medicaid. Inpatient and outpatient services rendered to Medicaid program beneficiaries are paid for on the basis of actual costs incurred. The Hospital is paid at a tentative rate with final settlement determined after submission of annual cost reports by the Hospital and audits thereof by the Medicaid fiscal intermediary. The Hospital's Medicaid cost reports have been audited by the Medicaid fiscal intermediary through December 31, 1991.

Blue Cross. Inpatient services rendered to Blue Cross subscribers under a local plan are paid for at prospectively determined rates per day of hospitalization. The prospectively determined per-diem rates are not subject to retroactive adjustment.

The Hospital has also entered into payment agreements with certain commercial insurance carriers, health maintenance organizations, and preferred provider organizations. The basis for payment to the Hospital under these agreements includes prospectively determined rates per discharge, discounts from established charges, and prospectively determined daily rates.

4. **Investment in Affiliated Entity.**

In 1993, the Hospital entered into an agreement with three unrelated hospitals to establish and operate an ambulatory care center. Each of the four hospitals invested $923,000 for a 25% equity interest in the common stock of the center. The investment by each hospital was $476,000 in 1993 and $447,000 in 1994, and the center began operations in 1993. The Hospital accounts for this investment by the equity method.

Summarized financial information from the financial statements of the ambulatory care center follows (dollar amounts in thousands):

	12/31/94	12/31/93
Current assets	$2,175	$1,708
Noncurrent assets	5,155	3,912
Current liabilities	1,710	1,320
Noncurrent liabilities	2,200	2,500
Stockholders' equity	3,420	1,800

	YEAR ENDED	
	12/31/94	12/31/93
Revenues	$3,850	$2,727
Net loss	(168)	(104)

5. **Assets Whose Use Is Limited.**

Assets whose use is limited that are required for obligations classified as current liabilities are reported as current assets. The composition of assets whose use is limited at December 31, 1994 and 1993 is indicated below (dollar amounts in thousands). Investments are stated at cost that approximates market.

	12/31/94	12/31/93
By board for acquisition of plant assets:		
Cash	$ 216	$ 307
Investments	6,184	8,593
Total	$ 6,400	$ 8,900

By agreements with third-party payors:		
Cash	$ 131	$ 96
Interest receivable	77	49
Investments	8,100	6,100
Total	$ 8,308	$ 6,245

Under malpractice funding arrangement—held by trustee:		
Cash	$ 72	$ 88
Investments	3,093	2,626
Total	$ 3,165	$ 2,714

Under indenture agreement—held by trustee:		
Cash	$ 127	$ 118
Investments	11,834	10,927
Interest receivable	86	63
Total	$12,047	$11,108

6. **Property, Plant, and Equipment.**

A summary of property, plant, and equipment at December 31, 1994 and 1993 follows (dollar amounts in thousands):

	12/31/94	12/31/93
Land	$ 2,600	$ 2,600
Land improvements	709	588
Buildings and improvements	42,456	41,977
Equipment	30,263	26,188
Equipment under capital leases	3,189	2,909
	79,217	74,262
Less accumulated depreciation	29,876	25,519
	49,341	48,743
Construction in progress	3,594	2,105
Property, plant, and equipment, net	$52,935	$50,848

Construction contracts of approximately $6,914,000 exist for remodeling of Hospital facilities. At December 31, 1994, the remaining commitment on these contracts approximated $3,320,000.

7. **Long-Term Debt and Capital Leases.**

A summary of long-term debt and capital leases at December 31, 1994 and 1993 follows (dollar amounts in thousands):

	12/31/94	12/31/93
8.75% Revenue Notes, due October 1, 2021, collaterized by a pledge of the Hospital's patient service revenues	$15,865	$17,460
9.00% Mortgage loan, due June 30, 2005, collaterized by a mortgage on property, plant, and equipment with an undepreciated cost of $8,525 at December 31, 1994	8,035	8,140
9.25% Notes payable, due April 1, 1999, unsecured	600	700
Total	24,500	26,300
Less current portion	750	900
Total long-term debt, net of current portion	$23,750	$24,500
Capital lease obligations, at varying rates of imputed interest from 10.25% to 12.75%, collateralized by leased equipment with a undepreciated cost of $1,100 at December 31, 1994	$ 881	$ 1,206
Less current portion	450	410
Capital lease obligations net of current portion	$ 431	$ 796

Under the terms of the Revenue Note Indenture, the Hospital is required to maintain certain deposits with a trustee. Such deposits are included in assets whose use is limited in the balance sheets. The Indenture also places limits on the incurrence of additional borrowings and requires that the Hospital satisfy certain measures of financial performance as long as the notes are outstanding.

Scheduled principal repayments on long-term debt and payments on capital lease obligations for the next five years are as follows (dollar amounts in thousands):

	Long-Term Debt	Obligations under Captial Leases
1995	$ 750	$ 410
1996	690	125
1997	650	125
1998	980	125
1999	1,030	96
	$4,100	881
Less amount representing interest on obligations under capital leases		81
		$ 800

A summary of interest cost and investment income on borrowed funds held by the trustee under the Revenue Note Indenture follows (dollar amounts in thousands):

	1994	1993
Interest cost:		
Capitalized	$ 643	$ 661
Charged to expenses	1,859	1,977
Total	$2,502	$2,638
Investment income:		
Capitalized	$ 427	$ 513
Credited to other revenues	311	346
Total	$ 738	$ 859

8. **Medical Malpractice Claims.**

The Hospital is uninsured with respect to medical malpractice risks. Losses from asserted claims and from unasserted claims identified under the Hospital's incident reporting system are accrued based on estimates that incorporate the Hospital's past experience, as well as other considerations including the nature of each claim or incident and relevant trend factors. Accrued malpractice losses have been discounted at rates ranging from 7.25 to 9.25 percent. No accrual for possible losses attributable to incidents that may have occurred, but that have not been identified under the incident reporting system, has been made because the amount is not reasonably estimable.

The Hospital has established an irrevocable trust fund for the payment of medical malpractice claim settlements. Professional insurance consultants have been retained to assist the Hospital with determining amounts to be deposited in the trust fund.

9. **Endowment Resources—Investments.**

Donor-restricted endowment resources in investment portfolios include marketable equity securities that are carried at the lower of aggregate cost or market. Marketable equity securities of endowment funds at December 31, 1994 and 1993 are summarized as follows (dollar amounts in thousands):

	1994	1993
Cost	$2,069	$1,836
Quoted market value	1,903	2,050
Gross unrealized gains	17	246
Gross unrealized losses	(183)	(32)

Realized gains (losses) on marketable equity securities of endowment funds amounted to $(440,000) in 1994 and $234,000 in 1993.

10. **Assets Held in Trust.**

The Hospital is an income beneficiary of the William Telkamp Kovener Trust. Because the assets of the trust are not controlled by the Hospital, they are not included in the Hospital's balance sheets. On December 31, 1994, the market value of the trust assets was approximately $1,874,200. Distributions of income are made at the discretion of the trustees. The income distributed to the Hospital by the trust is restricted for construction or equipment acquisitions, and amounted to $130,000 in 1994 and $110,000 in 1993.

11. **Related Party Transactions.**

Because of the existence of common trustees and other factors, the Hospital and Titera Health Foundation (Foundation) are related parties. The Foundation is authorized by the Hospital to solicit contributions on its behalf. In its general appeal for contributions to support the community's providers of healthcare services, the Foundation also solicits contributions for certain other health care entities. In the absence of donor restrictions, the Foundation has discretionary control over the amounts, timing, and use of its distributions.

Contributions made by the Foundation to the Hospital during the years ended December 31, 1994 and 1993 are reported in the Hospital's financial statements as follows (dollar amounts in thousands):

	1994	1993
Unrestricted contributions	$ 295	$ 430
Restricted contributions for:		
Specific operating purposes	250	175
Plant replacement and expansion	80	60

In addition, the Hospital made a capital contribution of $750,000 to Goodcare Health System in 1993.

12. Pension Plan.

The Hospital has a defined benefit pension plan covering substantially all of its employees. The plan benefits are based on years of service and the employees' compensation during the last five years of covered employment. The Hospital makes annual contributions to the plan equal to the amounts of net periodic pension cost. Contributions are intended to provide benefits attributed to service to date.

The actuarially computed net periodic pension costs for 1994 and 1993 included the following components (dollar amounts in thousands):

	1994	1993
Service cost-benefits earning during the period	$ 885	$ 804
Interest cost on projected benefit obligation	591	539
Actual return on plan assets	(860)	(770)
Net amortization and deferral	79	84
Net periodic pension cost	$ 695	$ 657

Assumptions used in the accounting for net periodic pension cost were as follows:

	12/31/94	12/31/93
Discount rates	6.8%	6.8%
Rates of increase in compensation levels	5.5	5.5
Expected long-term rate of return on assets	7.5	7.5

The pension plan's funded status and amounts recognized in the Hospital's balance sheets at December 31, 1994 and 1993 are indicated below (dollar amounts in thousands):

	1994	1993
Actuarial present value of benefit obligations:		
Vested benefit obligation	$ 7,512	$ 6,774
Nonvested benefit obligation	1,789	1,819
Accumulated benefit obligation	9,301	8,593
Effect of projected future compensation levels	928	880
Projected benefit obligation	10,229	9,473
Plan assets at fair value (primarily listed stocks and U.S. bonds)	10,375	9,560
Plan assets in excess of projected benefit obligation	146	87
Unrecognized net gain from past experience different from that assumed	(24)	(32)
Prior service cost not yet recognized in net periodic pension cost	51	63
Unrecognized net asset at January 1, 1993, being recognized over 15 years	(68)	(73)
Prepaid pension cost, included in other assets in the balance sheets	$ 105	$ 45

13. **Commitments.**

Leases that do not meet the criteria for capitalization are classified as operating leases with related rentals charged to operations as incurred. The following is a schedule, by year, of future minimum lease payments under operating leases at December 31, 1994 that have initial or remaining lease terms in excess of one year (dollar amounts in thousands):

Year Ending December 31	Minimum Lease Payments
1995	$ 422
1996	406
1997	381
1998	337
1999	305
Total	$1,851

Total rent expense in 1994 and 1993 for all operating leases was approximately $722,000 and $697,000, respectively.

14. **Functional Classification of Expenses.**

The Hospital's statements of income and other changes in unrestricted equity present expenses in a natural (object of expenditure) classification. Following is a functional classification of these expenses (after allocation of all indirect expenses) for the years ended December 31, 1994, and 1993 (dollar amounts in thousands):

	1994	1993
Nursing services	$36,717	$34,923
Other professional services	27,582	26,788
General services	17,379	16,840
Fiscal services	5,579	4,838
Administrative services	8,949	8,353
Research and education	2,524	2,295
Total expenses	$98,720	$94,047

15. Subsequent Event.

On February 11, 1995, the Hospital signed a contract in the amount of $2,916,000 for the purchase of certain real estate.

Index

About the Author

L. Vann Seawell has vast experience in financial accounting. A Professor Emeritus of Accounting in the Graduate School of Business at Indiana University, Dr. Seawell has published many books and monographys during the past 35 years. Among his efforts include *Hospital Financial Accounting Theory and Practice–Second Edition* (Healthcare Financial Management Association, 1987) and *Introduction to Hospital Accounting–Third Edition* (Healthcare Financial Management Association, 1992). From 1987 to 1993 Dr. Seawell was a member of the Healthcare Financial Management Association's Accounting Principles and Practices Board.

Dr. Seawell has a B.B.A. from Wake Forest University, an M.B.A. from Indiana University and a D.B.A. from Indiana University. He lives in Bloomington, Indiana.